ROCHESTER ADOLESCENT MEDICINE

Rochester Adolescent Medicine

The Journey Has Just Begun

Meghan E. Plog, MS
Elizabeth R. McAnarney, MD

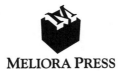

MELIORA PRESS

An imprint of the University of Rochester Press

First published 2024

Meliora Press is an imprint of the
University of Rochester Press
668 Mt. Hope Avenue, Rochester, NY 14620, USA
www.urpress.com

and Boydell & Brewer Limited
PO Box 9, Woodbridge, Suffolk IP12 3DF, UK
www.boydellandbrewer.com

ISBN-13: 978-1-64825-078-1

Library of Congress Cataloging-in-Publication Data

Names: Plog, Meghan E., author. | McAnarney, Elizabeth R., 1940– author.
Title: Rochester adolescent medicine : the journey has just begun / Meghan E. Plog, Elizabeth R. McAnarney.
Description: Rochester, NY : Meliora Press, an imprint of the University of Rochester Press, 2024.
Identifiers: LCCN 2023025979 | ISBN 9781648250781 (paperback; alk. paper)
Subjects: MESH: University of Rochester. Department of Pediatrics. Division of Adolescent Medicine. | Pediatricians | Faculty, Medical | Schools, Medical | Adolescent Medicine | New York | Biography
Classification: LCC RJ550 | NLM WZ 112.5.P3 | DDC 616.00835—dc23/eng/20231018
LC record available at https://lccn.loc.gov/2023025979

This publication is printed on acid-free paper.

Printed in the United States of America.

You know there must be ballast within the ship to make it go steady.

—Jeremiah Burroughs[1]

This volume is dedicated to Carole M. Berger, the "ballast of the Rochester Adolescent Medicine, Department of Pediatrics' ship." Her energy, creativity, kindness, and generosity have steadied our ship over nearly five decades. We extend our deepest gratitude for her remarkable service by dedicating this volume to her.

MEP/ERM

---

1 www.https:/teachingresources.org/2010/07/how-to-attain-contentment-by-jeremiah-burroughs/.

CONTENTS

PREFACE

The youth is the hope of the future.

—Jose Rizal[1]

Rochester Adolescent Medicine: The Journey Has Just Begun celebrates the Adolescent Medicine program at the University of Rochester (New York) Medical Center. During six decades, the program grew from a weekly ambulatory session to a fully functioning division of the Department of Pediatrics with an array of complex clinical, research, educational, and community programs of national/international significance.

In the pages that follow the reader will note the dedication and passion of the thirty-one featured former and present University residents, fellows, and faculty members to their chosen subspecialty of Adolescent Medicine. Their primary purpose is to help adolescents and their families be as healthy as possible as adolescents enter adulthood. They are fervent in their belief that "The youth is the hope of the future."

Ms. Meghan Plog has interviewed our colleagues to gain their perspectives and their insights into the effects of the program and its staff on the improvement of the health of adolescents, education of trainees, and contributions to new knowledge in Adolescent Medicine. We are very proud of the trainees who have graduated from our fellowship, established their professional independence, and significantly advanced the goals of excellence on behalf of adolescents, their families, and communities in national and international sites. They have truly spread the word about the evolving critical needs of adolescents all over the world. Many are still working in academic settings, schools, public health settings, and in adolescents' and families' homes. The

1 Jose Rizal Quotes. BrainyQuote.com. Brainy/Media Inc. 2023. https:/www.brainy quote.com/quotes/jose_rizal_244773, accessed April 10, 2023.

trainees featured in this volume are a small group chosen to represent the great number of practitioners whom we have trained over the decades.

The origins of adolescent health date back to the late 1700s; however, it was only recently, in the early 1950s, that modern practices of health care of adolescents began at Boston Children's Hospital with the creation of the Adolescent Unit, initially directed by J. Roswell Gallagher, MD. A history of the field of Adolescent Medicine is outlined by Dr. Felix P. Heald, a pioneer in the modern field of Adolescent Medicine, in the *Textbook of Adolescent Medicine* (1992).[2]

Early on in the growth of the subspecialty of Adolescent Medicine, the American Academy of Pediatrics (AAP) supported the efforts by a small group of national leaders to alert and educate health professionals about the importance of the care of adolescents and their families. The influence of the highly regarded AAP among pediatricians was seminal in providing legitimacy to Adolescent Medicine as a field.

The Society for Adolescent Medicine (SAM), now the Society for Adolescent Health and Medicine (SAHM), was established on April 28, 1968. A subspecialty board for Adolescent Medicine was approved in the early 1990s by the American Board of Pediatrics. Rochester faculty and fellows joined forces with their national colleagues as spokespersons for the burgeoning field.

Faculty and former fellows from Rochester Adolescent Medicine have been leaders at the forefront of almost every major decision about the field of Adolescent Medicine since its inception. In fact, several have led national and international organizations over the years. Five of our colleagues (Drs. Elster, Friedman, Kreipe, McAnarney, and Yancy) were presidents of SAHM. We believe that the five Rochester members leading SAHM represent the highest number of colleagues in one group in the country at the present time. All the more remarkable is that our program is relatively small.

Adolescent Medicine has never been more critical than it is now. We live in a deeply divided country where vulnerable citizens are scorned, bullied, and marginalized. The pioneers from decades ago had great foresight to create

---

2   Heald, Felix P. "The History of Adolescent Medicine." In *Textbook of Adolescent Medicine*, edited by Elizabeth R. McAnarney, Richard E. Kreipe, Donald P. Orr, and George D. Comerci, 1:1-5, Philadelphia, PA: W.B. Saunders Company, 1992.

the field of Adolescent Medicine and to continue its dedication to equity, diversity, and integrity in all programs.

With this book, we celebrate Rochester's six decades of contributions to optimum health for adolescents and their families. The Rochester, New York, community and the University of Rochester have been ideal partners in the creation of unique programs for adolescents and for training future generations of leaders in Adolescent Medicine.

The Department of Pediatrics at the University of Rochester has a long history of Community Pediatrics, led initially by Dr. Robert J. Haggerty. Our late founders of Rochester Adolescent Medicine, Drs. Stanford B. Friedman and Christopher H. Hodgman, were visionaries. Nationally, there were many supportive colleagues to whom we are indebted: Ms. Edie Moore, Drs. Robert Blum, Charles Irwin, Renée Jenkins, Marianne Felice, Michael I. Cohen, Iris Litt, Richard Brown, Richard Mackenzie, Joseph Rauh, Felix Heald, and Dale Garrell, representing a small number of leaders in the field of Adolescent Medicine. The lessons shared with and among these colleagues were important and prescient.

A special thank you to the Friedlander family for their support of the Adolescent Medicine program over the years.

We thank Donna Treat, Lauralee Haefner, and Ellyn Tarasuk for their contributions to the photographs in this volume. We also acknowledge Sonia Kane and Susan Smith of the University of Rochester Press for their contributions.

Carole M. Berger, to whom this book is dedicated, is the "ballast" of our ship. Carole has devoted forty-eight years of her life to administering programs in our Department of Pediatrics: the adolescent program for seventeen years, the chair's office in Pediatrics for thirteen years, and, for the past eighteen years, Dr. McAnarney's work. Her commitment, dedication, productivity, and optimistic consistency are all traits to be emulated.

Elizabeth R. McAnarney, MD
Distinguished University Professor
Chair Emerita, Department of Pediatrics
University of Rochester Medical Center
Department of Pediatrics/
Golisano Children's Hospital

ABBREVIATIONS

AAMC	Association of American Medical Colleges
AAP	American Academy of Pediatrics
ACE	Alliance for Clinical Education
ACGME	Accreditation Council for Graduate Medical Education
AMA	American Medical Association
APA	American Psychological Association
APD	Associate Program Director
APS	American Pediatric Society
AHEC	Area Health Education Centers
CDC	Centers for Disease Control
COMSEP	Council on Medical Student Education in Pediatrics
CRHI	Center for Rural Health Innovation
DIO	Designated Institutional Official
DSM	Diagnostic and Statistical Manual
ECHO	Extension for Community Health Care Outcomes
FNP	Family Nurse Practitioner
GME	Graduate Medical Education
GAPS	Guidelines for Adolescent Preventive Services
HIV	Human Immunodeficiency Virus
HRSA	Health Resources and Services Administration
ID	Infectious Diseases

IBM	International Business Machines
IUD	Intrauterine Device
LARC	Long-Acting Reversible Contraception
LEAH	Leadership Education in Adolescent Health
LEND	Leadership Education in Neurodevelopmental and Related Disabilities
MCHB	Maternal and Child Health Bureau
MPH	Master of Public Health
NIH	National Institutes of Health
NIMH	National Institute of Mental Health
NP	Nurse Practitioner
OBGYN	Obstetrics and Gynecology
PD	Program Director
PNP	Pediatric Nurse Practitioner
RAMP	Rochester Adolescent Maternity Program
RCSD	Rochester City School District
RGH/RRH	Rochester General Hospital/Rochester Regional Health
SAM	Society for Adolescent Medicine
SAHM	Society for Adolescent Health and Medicine
SBHCs	School-Based Health Centers
SMR	Sexual Maturity Ratings
TFA	Teach For America
UHS	University Health Service
UR	University of Rochester
URMC	University of Rochester Medical Center
URSMD	University of Rochester School of Medicine and Dentistry
WIC	Women, Infants, and Children

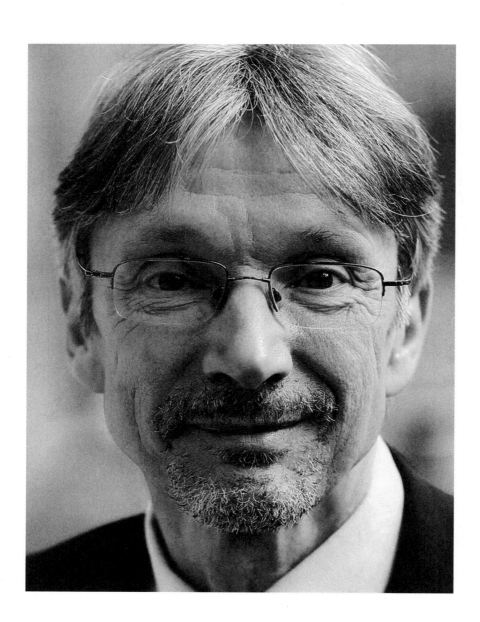

Chapter One

Frank M. Biro, MD

Frank Biro is a 1983 graduate of the University of Rochester combined Medicine-Pediatrics residency and received many of his earliest introductions to the field of adolescent medicine in Rochester. His successful career has included serving as the founding program director of the University of Cincinnati's Medicine-Pediatrics residency program, the director of the Division of Adolescent and Transition Medicine, and director of a robust research program. A prominent clinician and investigator, he has made significant contributions to the field.

Biro grew up in Allentown and Emmaus, Pennsylvania, without much exposure to higher education. His father attended school through sixth grade, his mother attended through ninth grade, and a few aunts and uncles completed high school, making Biro the first among his close relatives to pursue and obtain a college degree. After he received a congressional nomination to attend the Naval Academy in Annapolis, Maryland, he learned late in his senior year that he was color blind through failing the requisite color perception test, forcing him to pursue an alternative path for college at Drexel University. At Drexel, he joined nearly every professional organization and honor society, inadvertently creating quite a strong record of accomplishment for medical school. He had multiple teeth broken during a hockey game the week before his interview at Harvard Medical School, where he interviewed with Dr. Robert Masland, a prominent leader in the field of adolescent medicine ... and hockey fan. Fortunately, his appearance that day did not influence his acceptance negatively; he attended Harvard Medical School.

Biro was interested in primary care and originally planned to pursue internal medicine and pediatrics. His primary goal was to work with the Indian Health Service, where he had completed a medical school elective, before being encouraged by a mentor to pursue academic medicine instead. The competitive combined Medicine-Pediatrics program at the University of Rochester was recruiting only two residents that year. Dr. Biro remembers traveling to Rochester directly after a twenty-four-hour overnight call, driving through the following night and arriving thirty minutes before his interview. He remembers that it was snowing as he tried to find his way to Monroe Community Hospital to interview with a prominent rheumatologist, Dr. John Baum. "Some nice people directed me to where it was, and I went into his office and promptly fell asleep," he exclaimed. He remembers being awoken gently by Dr. Baum. He apologized profusely and explained it had been forty-eight hours since he had last slept. Dr. Baum was impressed that Biro carried on a cogent conversation for as long as he did on so little sleep and said, "You're the kind of guy we need here!" "And that's how I got to Rochester," he said, with a laugh.

Dr. Biro experienced a particularly influential moment as a resident when he had the opportunity to meet Dr. James Tanner, who popularized the use of the developmental "Tanner stages" system (now called Sexual Maturity Ratings [SMR]). Dr. Tanner was a visiting professor in the Department of Pediatrics at the University of Rochester, having been invited by Rochester's Dr. Gilbert B. Forbes. In need of someone to help chauffeur Dr. Tanner to his morning meetings and then back to the hotel at the end of each day, they asked Dr. Biro to help with this task, also inviting him to attend the dinners. Dr. Biro and Dr. Tanner had wonderful conversations during their times together and even began brainstorming postresidency training opportunities with Dr. Tanner in England, as Dr. Biro was interested in the developmental changes during puberty. "I wanted to be a junior James Tanner," he said. "But we never quite worked out the specifics of it—for instance, I failed to ask him about how much I would be paid for this opportunity," he said with a laugh. It turned out that the yearly stipend would be closer to a month's wage as a resident, and since Dr. Biro would technically be a foreign medical graduate, his additional economic opportunities would be limited. As a result, Dr. Biro pursued fellowship training in the States, but remained in contact with Dr. Tanner throughout the years, loosely collaborating, especially regarding his research. "When I came up with an idea, I would write a letter and float it by him; or when I would write a manuscript, I would send it to him and ask him what he thought about it. He was very gracious with his time and would write back, usually right away," Dr. Biro said. With a postresidency experience in England off the table, but his interest still piqued by adolescent development, Dr. Biro believed a fellowship in adolescent medicine would be a good fit and would allow him to center his career on puberty—a goal he has accomplished to the highest standards. In fact, while speaking at an international meeting approximately sixteen years ago, the host introduced him as "the new prince of puberty."

Already in his fourth year of residency, Biro made this decision to pursue fellowship training. It was late in the application cycle and Rochester had already secured their adolescent medicine fellow for the next year: Dr. David M. Siegel, a colleague and friend of Dr. Biro's. Interested in returning to Boston, Dr. Biro called Dr. Robert Masland only to learn that they had just sent out their fellowship offers. Dr. Masland assured him a position the following year, but as luck would have it, he called Dr. Biro back the next day with news that someone had declined, and offered that newly open position. "I had assumed that, like Rochester's fellowship program, it was a two-year fellowship, so imagine my surprise when I got there in July and found out it was only one year!" he said. "Since then, my life has been very organized and planned." Thus, just as soon as he began his fellowship, he was already on the search for his postgraduate position. There were only three open adolescent medicine faculty positions for that next year, and after he interviewed for two of them, he ultimately secured a job at Cincinnati Children's Hospital, where he would spend the remainder of his career.

While in Cincinnati, Dr. Biro cofounded the Medicine-Pediatrics residency program along with the director of Medicine and director of Pediatrics. Upon his own residency graduation, he and a few colleagues from Rochester and the University of North Carolina surveyed graduates on what they believed were the most and the least beneficial aspects of the training, and he was amazed at the consistency of responses across the different programs. He designed the curriculum in Cincinnati on the basis of that survey, publishing several papers on the findings as well. He served as the first residency director for nine years, as well as served two periods as the division chief of Adolescent Medicine. As chief, he said he always put his faculty and division first, something he witnessed Dr. Elizabeth McAnarney do in Rochester. He has also had an extremely successful research career with numerous major grants from the National Institutes of Health (NIH) and over 250 publications.

In fact, his research contributions remain among his proudest accomplishments. He describes his research as examining everyday issues and trying to establish evidenced-based norms for the practice of pediatrics and adult internal medicine. "Just because somebody said it was so, doesn't mean it should be," he said. "And so, I researched questions that people had assumed they all knew the answers to." One such project was the development of a training course for health care providers, teachers, counselors, and anyone who worked with adolescents, something he described as a "crash course on adolescence." He also remains proud of his clinical contributions, for which he credits his experience in Rochester for giving him a strong basis. "I worked really hard during residency, I enjoyed my time, and I enjoyed the people I worked with—both the residents and the faculty," he said. "I worked on my clinical skills to make myself as strong a clinician as I could, and Rochester really helped me do that." His clinical contributions have resulted in several much-deserved honors, including the notable Cincinnati Children's Hospital Clinical Care Achievement Award.

Throughout his career, he has witnessed changes in the field that have positively affected adolescents' health, including an increased awareness of issues such as gender health. Over the length of his career, he can remember from a time when he was learning about three or four transgender patients who were cared for at Johns Hopkins to ultimately working with Cincinnati's robust transgender program, which is one of the largest in the country and sees hundreds of patients. "I think we have developed an evidence-based approach for a lot of the things we do," he said. "And I think there is a healthy skepticism when somebody says, 'We do it because this is what we've always done.'" He added that subjects never considered previously are now openly discussed with a focus on destigmatization. He admits there is a long way to go, as many of the ills of adolescents are rooted in social issues—poverty, inadequate healthcare, limited education, poor housing, race, and food insecurity. "That's the last frontier, but it's going to be one of the toughest things to address," he said. "I think those are driving a lot of the issues and concerns. If as an adolescent you do not see a light at the end of the tunnel, it probably increases your likelihood of substance abuse, illegal activity, and other problems. We need to have salient education and meaningful opportunities for adolescents."

Dr. Biro has accomplished much in his career as a nationally and internationally acclaimed clinician, researcher, and educator. He has fond memories of his time in Rochester, where he gained experiences that helped him develop into the clinician and researcher he has become. His leadership, commitment to adolescent health, and important research questions that challenged assumptions and helped create evidence-based frameworks have all helped move the field forward in profound ways. Dr. Biro stands among a handful of academic investigators in adolescent medicine who have made substantive long-term contributions to our understanding of normal puberty and adolescence, and the health and social conditions that teens encounter. Throughout everything, Dr. Biro remains an empathic, kind, creative, and knowledgeable physician.

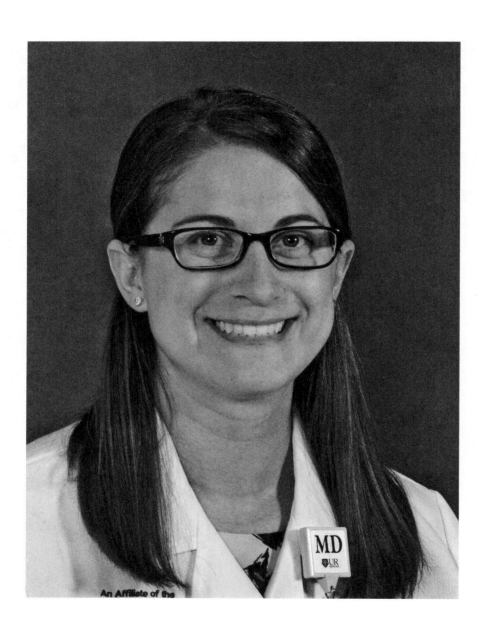

Chapter Two

ERICA A. BOSTICK, MD

With a background in internal medicine, Erica Bostick did not always plan for a career in adolescent medicine. However, the moment she was introduced to the field, she could not imagine herself doing anything else. Dr. Bostick graduated from the University of Rochester Adolescent Medicine Fellowship program in 2018 and joined the faculty as an assistant professor immediately after her fellowship. Her unique background and interests have brought new insight and collaborations to the division and fellowship program, contributing greatly to its services and educational offerings.

Bostick grew up in Central New Jersey. While her father is a dentist, she says she never felt any pressure to pursue the medical field. She dreamed of a city college experience, and following her New York City–raised parents' advice to start with a smaller big city, she attended Northeastern University in Boston, Massachusetts. She has the fondest memories of her undergraduate years, particularly appreciating her school's unique co-op program. She pursued two co-ops, which provided her working experiences in research labs through Harvard University and their partnering hospitals, and led her to pursue a major in medical laboratory science. "My clinical rotations plus my co-ops really had me curious about the patient side of the sample I was receiving, running, or studying," she said, and she set her sights on medical school with the eventual goal of pursuing infectious diseases (ID).

After experiencing initial challenges, Bostick looked for a less traditional pathway to becoming a physician and attended American University of the Caribbean in St. Maarten. She completed her first two basic science years on the island, followed by clinical rotations throughout the world—from London to Miami to New York City. She reflects that although it was a different path than she had originally envisioned taking, she says, "It really gave me the opportunity to not only try out different fields of medicine during my clinical years, but also in different locations and different countries, so it was really an enriching experience."

On July 1, 2013, Dr. Bostick began her internal medicine residency at St. Luke's/Roosevelt Hospital (now Mount Sinai Morningside and Mount Sinai West) in New York City, and on July 2, 2013, took her first on-call—an abrupt start that she describes as a bit traumatizing. While she had the support of her family forty miles away, the constant high volume and high acuity in this setting were shocking and overwhelming. However, thanks to this high volume, she had significant exposure to the field of ID, but ended up beginning to feel that it was not something she could see herself doing forever. She was drawn to the aspects of human immunodeficiency virus (HIV) medicine, sexually transmitted infections (STIs), and sexual and reproductive health, but realized that this niche would not lead to a typical career in ID. "I remember so vividly walking from one hospital to another, which was ninety blocks, on a beautiful day and having this very clichéd existential crisis moment of, 'I just did all this stuff for the last decade and now I'm totally lost. What am I going to do?'" she said.

As she walked, she thought deeply about her interests and found herself returning to sexual and reproductive health and empowerment of body autonomy. These interests were first formed while she was in college and served as a volunteer with the Peer Health Exchange, providing peer health education in inner city Boston schools, and were further fostered in residency through time spent working on HIV service. Drawn to the content and the adolescent population, she did some research and learned that adolescent medicine would be a path that would allow for these interests to be cultivated and practiced. She quickly lined up electives at neighboring institutions, Columbia and Montefiore, where she says she "found my people."

"I just loved the energy and loved the passion that all of the adolescent medicine doctors had. We were all in it for the same reason—all about empowering teens at such a critical time of their life," she said. "There were components of primary care and components of pediatrics that scared me," she admits, "but I really found hope in medicine again." She connected with her local New York chapter of the Society for Adolescent Health and Medicine (SAHM), further solidifying her realization that this was where she belonged.

As she interviewed throughout the country for her fellowship, she said she didn't know if her background in internal medicine would work for or against her. As she interviewed in Rochester, she hoped it would be the former, as she said, "I completely fell in love with the team and program. I had no idea such a program existed—culture wise, people wise, or medicine wise." She was thrilled to join the group and embarked on a two-year fellowship, the length required by the American Board of Internal Medicine (ABIM). She remembers being assured that this would be enough time by program director Dr. Susan "Shellie" Yussman, whom Dr. Bostick says she trusts implicitly. "She believed in me—it meant so much to me for her to see me as the person that I am," she said. "And that's really the sense I got immediately interviewing in Rochester and then staying on as a fellow and working with everyone within the division and department, and even outside of the department. People care about you for you as a person and a doctor; and not just how you look on paper." She spent two years training in adolescent medicine, from caring for her first ever eating disorder and transgender patients, to graduating feeling well supported, mentored, and prepared to take care of the full spectrum of patients within the field.

As graduation and her job search approached, she found herself weighing factors of geographical proximity to family, the fact that she and her husband had a small child and one more on the way, and realized, "In reality, I don't ever want to leave this place!" She cherished the work she was doing, the people she worked with, and the Rochester community she was serving. "It was worth it enough to me to be a little further from my family to have a leader like Shellie and to have colleagues like all of my colleagues. It's just a one in a million chance," she said. She appreciated the culture in Rochester, which she describes as very community focused and encouraging of community engagement, as well as self-reflective and committed to improvement. Fortunately, the division was hiring and Dr. Bostick interviewed and was offered the position.

As she worked to define her areas of interest, she was able to narrow them down to contraception and sexual and reproductive healthcare. During her fellowship training, she had the opportunity to complete an STI Intensive offered through the Monroe County Department of Health's Sexually Transmitted Diseases (STD) Clinic, which solidified these interests for her. She found the STD Clinic to be an incredible place and appreciated the unique local relationship between Monroe County and the University of Rochester (UR), as the clinic is fully staffed by UR employees. "The people there are so wonderful and so dedicated to the community," she said. "After two days there, I thought, 'These people are amazing and I need to be here!'—just like how I felt when interviewing for adolescent medicine fellowship." She felt so strongly about her interest to continue her work there that she tracked down the director, Dr. Margie Urban, to introduce herself as a soon-to-be fellowship graduate and new faculty member. As fate would have it, it turns out Dr. Bostick didn't stray too far from her initial interest in infectious diseases, as Dr. Urban, an adult ID physician, has become a key mentor for her. Dr. Bostick spends time each month working at the STD Clinic and collaborates with Dr. Urban on grants and educational talks, which have given her regional, statewide, and national exposure. "I feel like I've contributed to the dissemination of some really important information," she said. "It has really challenged me, for the good of myself, the work and the good of others, and has created a lot of opportunities for me."

This partnership has also created significant opportunities for the fellowship program. Through Dr. Bostick's aid, the STD Clinic is now an official rotation for all adolescent medicine fellows and provides substantial gynecological exposure, an area in which the fellowship program was looking to grow. Dr. Bostick has also greatly contributed to fellow involvement in the division's quality improvement (QI) efforts. She now partners with all first-year fellows on their QI project, giving them early opportunities to practice and cultivate these skills, including presenting at the local, regional, or national level, all while completing meaningful projects for the division, department, and hospital.

However, when reflecting on what she is most proud of, she says, "I'm most proud of, in general, the work that we do, the way we do it, and the people I work with. I truly feel like I have a work family—we have each other's backs and we really deliver critical services to a very large population. … And we take that really seriously and collectively prioritize patient care, but we also prioritize our family and our work-life balance." While an institutional and even larger national awareness of work-life balance has been growing, Dr. Bostick says the adolescent medicine group was ahead of the curve in that prioritization. "I'm just most proud of our mentality and the work that we do. I really think the leadership we have within the division and the dedication we have to our patients and each other is something that stands out to me about the Division of Adolescent Medicine at the University of Rochester."

From her time in fellowship, she has already witnessed changes in the field. One such area that she has found herself involved in is that of adolescent confidentiality and the risks posed as technology increases. There is a recognition for necessary system changes, and Dr. Bostick looks forward to continuing to advocate and help make improvements in that arena. She has also witnessed improvement in workflows and practices made from reflection through the critical lens of health equity, inequality, and systemic racism. "We are really trying to identify the patients that need us the most and think about how we can get to them and get them to us," she said. "We are constantly reevaluating ourselves as adolescent medicine providers, based on internal feedback, external feedback from patients, colleagues, whoever, and we try to implement and incorporate their suggestions. I think adolescent medicine in Rochester is able to problem solve creatively and collaboratively to make things happen even if there are barriers."

Dr. Bostick's passion for the betterment of adolescent health and the ever-evolving field of adolescent medicine is evident in all she undertakes. Her unique background and interests have built collaborations that have greatly contributed to the division's missions, and her commitment to advocacy and providing equitable care are quintessential to moving the field forward.

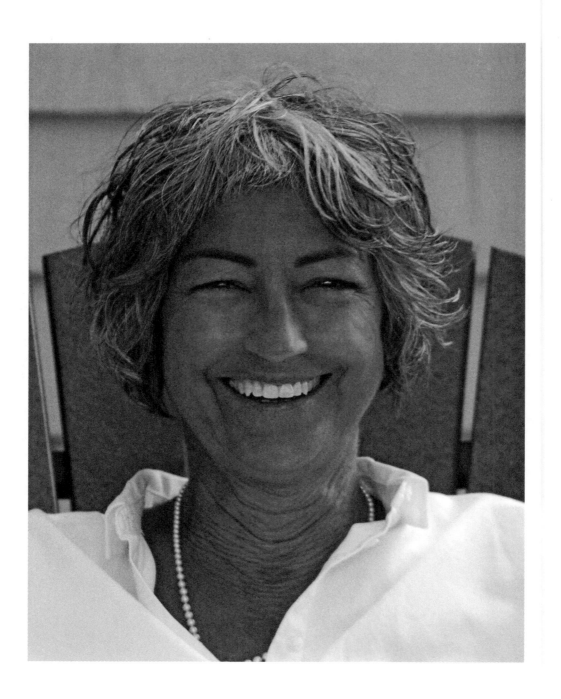

Chapter Three

SUZANNE J. BUMPUS, RN, MS, FNP-C

Suzanne Bumpus has been involved with Rochester's Adolescent Medicine program throughout her career, from nursing student to registered nurse to nurse practitioner, and in inpatient, ambulatory, and University Health settings. Her passion for and the ease with which she works with adolescents has been instrumental in the lives of her many patients, the division, and the broader community.

A Rochester native, Bumpus grew up in Fairport, New York, and was the oldest of three children to parents who were immigrants. She did not have much exposure to the medical field growing up and nursing was not her first path, but rather a field she said she entered "in a back-door kind of way." After graduating from Fairport High School, she attended Rochester Institute of Technology (RIT) to pursue a degree in social work. Finding that the program was not a good fit, she left and began working for a county-funded social services program, the Youth Employment Training Program (YETP), which provided working experience for under-resourced adolescents. While Suzanne enjoyed this work, she said it felt like a Band-Aid rather than a more permanent solution, as there was not much accountability on the part of the employer or the adolescent. It was during that time that she began to think nursing might be a better option for her. Changes in life circumstances left her a single parent and necessitated a more aggressive approach to employment. With the support of her parents and multiple odd jobs, she began full-time nursing school at the University of Rochester's School of Nursing.

While originally thinking she would pursue labor and delivery nursing, everything changed when she began her pediatrics rotation on 4-1400, the adolescent floor (this was during the time when the units of the children's hospital were separated by developmental age, rather than by medical specialty). While most of the students in her cohort were interested in working with the infants/toddlers, she said working on 4-1400 felt like being home. "I did my rotation there and thought, 'Oh my, this is my perfect fit,'" she said. While she may have had that "aha" moment during her clinical rotations, she said if she looks back historically, this was always the age-group she most enjoyed—whether interacting with the adolescent volunteers for her children's Brownie troops when she served as a leader or providing adolescents work experiences through her first job with YETP. She laughs, saying that her husband will agree that she is an adolescent at heart. Upon her nursing school graduation, she was hired on the adolescent floor, which she says was a perfect introduction into her nursing career.

She served as a nurse in the adolescent unit for four and one-half years before she remarried and her family moved to Canandaigua, New York, necessitating a job closer to home. With a lack of pediatric options in that area, she found herself caring for patients at the other end of the spectrum—long-term care for patients who had dementia at Thompson Health in Canandaigua. "I loved that too," she said. "It fit my needs at the time." After a few years, the hospital reinstated their tuition reimbursement program, allowing for one class each semester. She decided to enroll in a graduate course at St. John Fisher University—if she liked it, she would continue. She ended up loving it and spent the next five years earning her master's degree as a family nurse practitioner (FNP). Since she knew her true calling was working with adolescents, she sought out opportunities for clinical rotations at the health centers of RIT and Marshall High School, and at Planned Parenthood. "I arranged my clinical time in places that I felt would best meet my needs and perhaps an employment opportunity would emerge," she said. However, the fateful moment that a door ended up opening was at a Rochester Philharmonic Concert at CMAC (an area performing arts center in Canandaigua). She and her husband met Dr. Richard Kreipe, the University of Rochester Adolescent Medicine division chief at the time, and his wife, Dr. Mary Sue Jack, who was one of Ms. Bumpus's professors in nursing school. After catching up, Dr. Kreipe offered her a per diem job with the division while their nurse practitioner was out on leave, allowing her to work a few days a week that summer; when Dr. Kreipe eventually secured additional funding, she joined them full-time.

During her eight years as a nurse practitioner in the division, she worked in both inpatient and ambulatory capacities—seeing patients at East High School, working in the Teen-Tot clinic, and becoming involved with the Leadership Education in Adolescent Health (LEAH) program, as both a fellow and preceptor. She took care of patients who had eating disorders, anxiety, and depression, and provided contraceptive counseling. During this time, she learned to place intrauterine devices (IUDs) and NEXPLANON, procedures that she continues to perform in her current position. Her role in bringing the nursing perspective and serving as a liaison between the adolescent medicine faculty and nurses on the adolescent inpatient unit is what she believes was one of her greatest contributions, as well as the education she provided to the nurses. As part of their orientation, new nurses were required to spend an afternoon observing care in the ambulatory setting. "Providing them with a different perspective on care for this population enhanced their insight when inpatient care was necessary," she said.

After her time spent in the Division of Adolescent Medicine, Ms. Bumpus began working in a similar capacity in her role as a nurse practitioner with University Health Service (UHS) on Rochester's undergraduate campus, a position from which she recently retired. Interestingly, three of the providers at UHS had an adolescent medicine background. "We were well-represented there," she said with a smile. Although it is officially primary care, she cared for patients who had eating disorders and provided contraceptive services, skills she acquired while working in adolescent medicine. She provided education through campus outreach/student programming and interacted with the adolescent medicine fellows who spent time rotating at UHS. She has continued to be involved in the Society for Adolescent Health and Medicine (SAHM), including program planning and serving on the Governance Review Committee. She remains grateful for Dr. Kreipe's mentorship and credits her time in adolescent medicine for many of the opportunities that came her way, including involvement in research, speaking opportunities, and developing test questions for pediatric nursing certification (PNC). "I have loved what I've done, have met some fabulous people, and ultimately have grown as a provider," she said.

She has seen the field grow and evolve since her first position as an RN in 1993, noting that she has witnessed an increased awareness and cognizance of the fact that there is a transition period between childhood and adulthood, and that there are specialists trained to provide that kind of care. "Our society in general has recognized there is this gap, resulting in adolescents receiving more services. A great example is the development of entities such as Rochester's Complex Care Center that provides transition care for adolescents who have chronic illnesses," she said. She has seen the division change as a result of these needs through expanded services in reproductive health and gender health care. As for the future, she believes it will greatly depend on the individual needs of adolescents, but envisions a need for more mental health services to combat the effects of the COVID-19 pandemic that reduced interaction with peers, something that was felt acutely on the undergraduate campus.

Ms. Bumpus has accomplished much in her career while also raising a family—in fact, it was her role as a mother, but also feeling like an adolescent at heart, that she believes uniquely enabled her to relate to both patient and parent, allowing her to help bridge the gap when needed. When reflecting on what she is most proud of, she said, "I think I'm just living proof that you can teach an old dog new tricks," remarking that she finished her bachelor's degree at thirty-six years old as a single parent of two children, and went on to receive her master's degree at age fifty. "I've ticked off things that I never thought I would do," she said, including getting her master's degree, contributing to the body of knowledge through research publications, speaking at and conference planning, and chairing and serving on committees for the Pediatric Nursing Conference and SAHM.

She credits her time in adolescent medicine for allowing much of this to come to fruition. "That's where I developed as a nurse and as a provider, learning all the time and honing my skills as a practitioner," she said. "It helped me to identify what I was really passionate about. I think it has helped me be who I am, to be a better provider." Former Adolescent Medicine division chief and

Department of Pediatrics Chair Emerita Dr. Elizabeth McAnarney has served as a role model to her. "She loves what she does, she's passionate about her work, and she makes everybody around her feel important and wanting to emulate the characteristics that make her such a kind, good provider and caring person," Ms. Bumpus said. "She's an amazing woman, and I've been so privileged to have her be a part of my life and my career."

Ms. Bumpus's contributions to the Division of Adolescent Medicine, Rochester community, and field of adolescent health have been varied and impactful. She is a true testament to following your passion and making those dreams a reality, and Rochester has surely benefited from being on the other side of that passion.

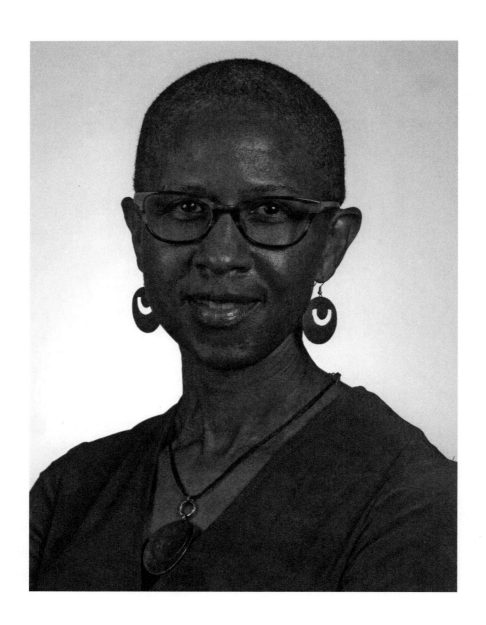

Chapter Four

ADRIENNE STITH BUTLER, PhD

Adrienne Stith Butler is a prominent psychologist and expert in science policy who has held leadership roles within the National Academies of Sciences, Engineering, and Medicine and the American Psychological Association (APA). Part of her professional journey took place at the University of Rochester when she served as a pediatric psychology fellow and Leadership Education in Adolescent Health (LEAH) fellow from 1997 to 1999. Her involvement in the Division of Adolescent Medicine's interdisciplinary LEAH training program provided her with experiences and skills that she has utilized throughout her career in public policy.

Stith Butler grew up in a military family, although instead of making frequent moves, they were permanently stationed at West Point where her father was a physics professor. She attended Johns Hopkins University for her undergraduate education, entering as a biophysics major. However, during her sophomore year, she wanted to change course. Feeling unsure of what direction to go, she went to the academic advising office and took a career aptitude test. "They told me, 'You would be a perfect psychologist,' so I said, 'Great, sign me up!'" she said with a smile. She changed her major and began volunteering at the Johns Hopkins Hospital's Kennedy Krieger Institute, a center for children and young adults with developmental disabilities. She found much fulfillment and continued to work at the institute throughout her undergraduate time, including summers, and obtained a job there upon graduation.

When applying to graduate programs in psychology, Stith Butler was drawn to the University of Vermont for the work they were doing with treatment in community settings. "It was during the time when they were closing institutions and placing kids in communities and wrapping services around them, so that was super exciting and I was thrilled I got in there," she said. She was able to research and interview families about their satisfaction with services, as well as participate in clinical work. She completed her pre-doctoral internship at Children's Memorial Hospital in Chicago, Illinois where she received her first introduction to pediatric psychology. "I had a lot of different experiences that year and the one that really resonated with me was pediatric psychology and the consultation services I did on the medical floors," she said. Interested in furthering that education, she applied for a postdoctoral fellowship in pediatric psychology at the University of Rochester and while interviewing, learned of the Division of Adolescent Medicine's LEAH program.

The University of Rochester was one of seven institutions in the nation to receive funding from the Maternal and Child Health Bureau (MCHB) for its LEAH program, which provided leadership training to graduate and postgraduate trainees within five core disciplines—medicine, nursing, nutrition, psychology, and social work. Drawn to the program's interdisciplinary focus, Adrienne signed on to complete two postdoctoral experiences in Rochester—one in pediatric psychology and one as a LEAH fellow. "I remember my LEAH year very well," she said. "It was the first time I really had immersive experiences with people from different disciplines." She reflects that her previous experiences in psychology were more siloed—consisting of going to the hospital for consultations and then returning back to her office in a separate psychology building. However, with LEAH, "we were all in it together," she said. When she thinks of the program and of Rochester Adolescent Medicine, she says, "I think about the commitment to interdisciplinary and comprehensive care, which may be more common now, but at the time, that really wasn't anything I had experienced before."

The LEAH program also provided her with more exposure to research and opportunities to teach, specifically a statistics class for her LEAH colleagues, something she had never done before. "It was a really great experience in making me think about things I could do other than providing direct psychology services," she said. In fact, she credits much of her experience as a LEAH fellow with inspiring her to pursue policy, as she found that many of the psychology-related issues she encountered were part of larger systemic problems. "I really do credit the experience during that time to my feeling that I wanted to tackle problems from a different angle," she said.

With her sights set on policy, she moved to Washington, DC, for a fellowship through the APA as a public policy scholar where she lobbied on Capitol Hill around issues including student services in schools and health inequities. She then began working at the Institute of Medicine at the National Academy of Sciences, a government chartered not-for-profit institution founded by President Lincoln to advise the government on matters of science (which has since grown to include additional disciplines). She held various roles within the institute, ultimately serving as associate director and then director of the Board on Behavioral, Cognitive, and Sensory Sciences within the Division of Behavioral and Social Sciences and Education.

Much of Dr. Stith Butler's work consisted of convening panels of experts to help answer questions that came from agencies or congressional mandates, and producing technical reports with the findings. She ran studies on topics ranging from preparing for terrorism, to setting an agenda for preterm birth research, to end of life care, to the future of nursing, to evaluating the Title X family planning program. She said the most important part was assembling the right group of people. "It wasn't just 'What experts do you need to answer a question?' but 'What combination of expertise do you need?'" They placed much emphasis on diversification of the discipline area, as well as on diversity of age, gender, race, ethnicity, and geographic location of experts in order to get the richest product possible. "It was a huge swath of work all intended to help inform where fields should go, where resources should go, and what research should be pursued," she said. "It was super satisfying work intellectually and a very interesting use of psychology skills."

Throughout these processes, Stith Butler found herself drawing from skills she learned and experiences she garnered through her time as a LEAH fellow, including a strong education in adolescent health leadership and research in an environment of interdisciplinary teamwork. Something she remains most proud of is her ability to work collaboratively across disciplines, which became extremely helpful in her work convening multidisciplinary panels.

Further, she found herself tapping into previous experiences in the field of adolescent medicine for many of her projects, particularly those pertaining to preterm birth and family planning, both of which greatly affect the adolescent population. However, even for topics that did not appear to overtly affect adolescents, she found she was able to view them through a unique lens and bring that important perspective to the table. "The LEAH program gave me more of a holistic lens," she said. "I have lots of fond memories of that time, the impact of that work, and how it helped to point me in this direction."

After spending over twenty years at the National Academy of Sciences, Dr. Stith Butler was offered a position at the APA in October 2021 as the Deputy Chief Science Officer. She helps lead the APA's initiative to increase the footprint of psychological sciences within the organization—a vast field that includes, for example, cognitive, developmental, and neuroscience components—as well as helping educate the public about what psychological science is and the impact it has on everyone's lives. This became especially critical during the COVID-19 pandemic, as Stith Butler reports that psychologists have become among the most recruited experts for news stories—covering topics including vaccine hesitancy and how youth are coping during the pandemic. "There is so much about psychological science that we want to make known," she said, and her role is helping make that happen. "It has been great to return to psychology, but with this really interesting lens about all that science does for society, and trying to think about how scientists and associations in their silos can think about the problems that need to be solved in society," she said.

Dr. Stith Butler has spent her career as a strong leader and advocate for change, making significant contributions to initiatives that affect the whole population, inclusive of adolescents. Her unique background that includes training in leadership and adolescent health has given her important insight as she has worked to improve systemic and public policy issues on the national stage.

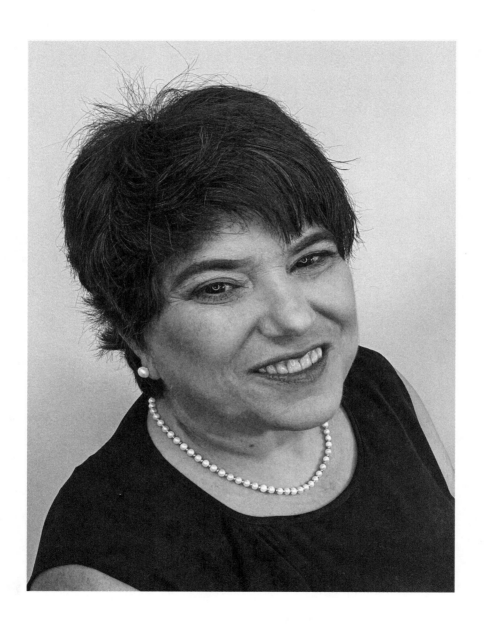

Chapter Five

Giuseppina "Giosi" Di Meglio, MD, MPH, FRCP, FSAHM

A 1997 graduate of the Adolescent Medicine Fellowship program and a 1998 graduate with her Master of Public Health (MPH) degree, Giuseppina "Giosi" Di Meglio has led a fruitful career as a true advocate in adolescent health. A key participant in the pursuit of achieving recognition of adolescent medicine as an official subspecialty in Canada, as well as a champion in the ongoing fight for no-cost and confidential contraception for adolescents, she has made a significant impact in the lives of adolescents and those training to become specialists—pushing boundaries and moving the field forward.

Di Meglio is a first-generation Canadian, born in Montreal to parents who emigrated from Italy just two years prior to her birth. "My parents really valued education, but neither one of them was educated," she said. Her father finished second grade and her mother finished fifth grade. "So, I was little out in left field going through the educational pathway." She received her bachelor's degree from Concordia University in Canada, following which her interest in science led her to brief stints as a PhD student and a high school science teacher in Harlem, New York. Realizing she had not quite found her calling in the classroom, but interested in finding a way to still work with children and make a difference, she pursued the route of adolescent medicine after meeting her school's physician, who shared insights on her own career path.

Interested in returning to Canada, Di Meglio attended medical school at Memorial University of Newfoundland, which she says was a "stupendous fit." With a small class size of forty-eight students, she feels fortunate for the flexibility and experiences that afforded—for instance, with minimal specialty and subspecialty training at the institution, medical students had much hands-on exposure working with patients. She originally envisioned a career in obstetrics and gynecology with an emphasis on the care of adolescents. "But as I was thinking about what I wanted to do and how I wanted to do it, I came to the philosophical understanding that by the time they were going to be seeing an obstetrician-gynecologist, it was a little late in the game," she said. "I wanted to be able to do something before that, to be involved with care before that." In determining her path to adolescent medicine, she ultimately decided on residency training in pediatrics, as she wanted to choose a specialty that would allow official certification in the subspecialty (which at the time was only pediatrics and internal medicine). After marrying an American whose career would take them back to the United States, she completed her pediatric residency in New York City at Montefiore Medical Center.

"I surprised myself because I thought, 'I'm just going to slog my way through this and get to where I can work with adolescents,' but I ended up really liking to work with little kids!" she said. This is something she attributes to her program director—a phenomenal pediatrician who taught her much about working with children and doing it well. However, she knew her end goal was still to pursue adolescent medicine fellowship so that she could work with adolescents as much as possible. She had her first child exactly four weeks before residency graduation and took her baby on the interview trail with her, including to Rochester. "I really loved the people there, and I was really excited by the work that they had been doing with pregnant teens," she said. "And so, I chose to come to Rochester, and the rest is history!"

Dr. Di Meglio looks back on her training in Rochester fondly—particularly remembering the clinical research that created an exciting and intellectually stimulating environment, which helped foster her niche research on adolescent breastfeeding. She was always interested in the research questions that asked "How are we going to help do this better" and "How do we improve things for people?" Thus, mentored by Dr. Jonathan Klein, Dr. Ruth Lawrence, and Dr. Cindy Howard, and using the Rochester Adolescent Maternity Program (RAMP) as her laboratory, she designed an intervention that paired peer mentors with young women who decided to breastfeed to serve as support coaches. Although there were difficulties and barriers that they encountered, they were ultimately able to enroll and provide support to almost one hundred adolescents.

She notes that the intellectual environment in Rochester is the most vibrant she has experienced in her career—from the consistent weekly forums to discuss clinical research and the collaboration, coaching, and support provided, to the forward-thinking spirit and attitude that focused on how to deliver healthcare more broadly and equitably. This latter aim was achieved through partnerships with a local community health system, Rochester General Hospital/Rochester Regional Health (RGH/RRH), as well as local clinics such as the Anthony Jordan Health Center—partnerships that aimed to provide better access to care. "I feel really privileged to have had the opportunity to train in Rochester," she said. "We were the beneficiaries of that attitude and that forward thinking spirit and that kind of political movement." Even though those partnerships had been forged prior to her time there, she said, "That environment continued—that sense of 'We've got to figure out how to do this better' and 'We're in it for everyone.' There was that vibe that was really quite energizing. It was a unique medical/intellectual environment."

However, perhaps one of her fondest recollections of her time in Rochester is Dr. Elizabeth McAnarney's personal interest and mentorship of the adolescent medicine fellows even after she became chair of the Department of Pediatrics. In fact, Dr. McAnarney's career guidance remains one of her greatest memories, and she often finds herself quoting Dr. McAnarney in her interactions with her own trainees. Dr. McAnarney's advice of breaking apart decision-making into manageable pieces, such as five-year increments, gave Dr. Di Meglio the permission to make decisions with both her family and career in mind. She said: "It really freed me to make choices that helped me to have time to spend with my family. I had little kids and I wanted to be able to be present for their growth, and to not feel like that meant that I was giving up research forever, or that I had to compromise on family life in order to start building a career, or that I had to make the exact right decision and it had to be a decision that was going to fit the rest of my life." It was advice that she was very grateful for, and has helped her throughout her career.

Following fellowship, Dr. Di Meglio and her family spent three years on the West Coast, where she served as the medical director for the Kent Teen Clinic in in Kent, Washington, an adolescent health consultant for the Seattle-King's County Public Health Department where she oversaw ten school-based health centers, as well as took time off to spend with her children. After deciding they would like to be closer to family on the East Coast, she and her spouse agreed to move wherever one of them first secured a job, which led them back to Canada at Montreal Children's Hospital, where she has been for over twenty years.

Between 2005 and 2007, Dr. Di Meglio was actively involved in the process of securing official recognition of adolescent medicine as a subspecialty of pediatrics in Canada, a recognition by the Royal College of Physicians and Surgeons of Canada that took place in the spring of 2007. Following that acceptance, she created an accredited fellowship program at Montreal Children's where she continues to serve as the program director.

Another passion of hers is socialized medicine and the movement to include pharmaceutical coverage among the covered benefits. "It's all fine and good to have access to the medical care, but if you can't afford the medicine, you're still in a difficult position," she said. In particular, she is helping lead the way in fighting for confidential, no-cost access to all forms of contraception for adolescents and young adults, something that is not uniformly available in Canada. She served as the lead author for the Canadian Pediatric Society's position statement stating that all adolescents should have access to no-cost contraception confidentially. "I think it's an important conversation and something we have to make happen," she said. "We shouldn't be waiting until we're having the conversation about what to do when you have a mistimed pregnancy; we should be trying to deliver the most effective contraception to young people who do not want to be pregnant, and making contraception accessible and available so that people can make that choice. The position statement was an important milestone and I'm hoping to continue to move that agenda forward."

Dr. Di Meglio has seen the field grow and evolve throughout her time in practice. "I'm in the middle of my third decade of practice and in that time, I've seen us really change the way we approach adolescents and their families in very positive ways," she said. "I think the adolescent medicine of thirty years from now will probably be very different from the way we practice today," she said, noting that both social media and the COVID-19 global pandemic have "changed the game in many ways." Through these changes, she said it remains important to have people interested and invested in adolescents, including through fellowship-trained specialists, and even beyond. "I think there are a lot of people out there caring for adolescents in very wonderful, compassionate ways, and that's really what we need," she said. "But I think that there's definitely unmet needs for providers who are interested in championing kids. They do not need to be people who are doing adolescent medicine all the time, but just caring about adolescents and understanding how to reach them and how to help them without enabling them. I think that we need many, many, many more people than we'll ever train in adolescent fellowship programs to be present for teenagers." An important way for this to be accomplished, she says, is through the field maintaining a presence in training centers so that the maximum number of trainees gain some exposure in working with adolescents effectively.

Dr. Di Meglio has accomplished much in her career, including leading major efforts that have significant influence in the lives and health of adolescents, the careers of medical trainees, and the field as a whole. It is work to which she continues to devote her time and passionate energy; as she says, "I'm hoping that my biggest contribution hasn't quite happened yet." While she knows her work is not done, her advocacy and work for positive change have certainly left their mark. Dr. Di Meglio's optimism, creativity, and productivity have influenced the field of adolescent medicine internationally and nationally.

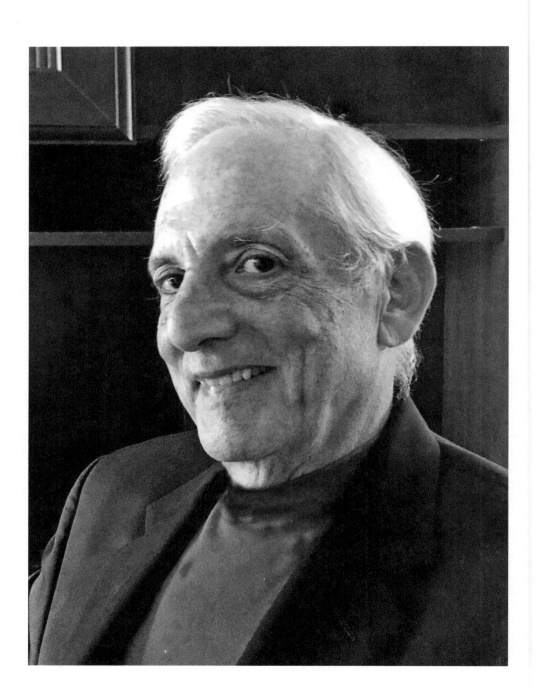

Chapter Six

ARTHUR B. ELSTER, MD, MJ

Arthur Elster has been an advocate for adolescent health for over forty years. From developing multiple national programs in adolescent medicine, to becoming a leader at the American Medical Association (AMA), to his most recent work teaching public health policy as it relates to adolescents, he has led the field forward in remarkable ways. A 1979 graduate of the Rochester Adolescent Medicine Fellowship program, he is grateful for the start in his career it provided him and attributes many of his successes to what he learned through those early experiences.

Elster grew up on the southeast coast of Texas in Port Arthur and believes a formative part of his history was growing up Jewish in what he experienced as a religiously intolerant and racist part of the country—both of which he witnessed firsthand. He graduated from Tulane University and received his medical degree from the University of Texas Medical Branch in Galveston. The years of his formal education were during a tumultuous era in American history when many citizens were fighting for social justice, including issues about civil rights and gender equality. The now historic Roe v. Wade case also occurred, which focused on changing abortion laws. "There was a lot of activism," he said. "And there was a lot of feeling that there were things that needed to be done." His interest in adolescent medicine was sparked during medical school when he spent a summer rotating at Letterman Army Medical Center in San Francisco, witnessing firsthand the Oakland riots and the flower children's movement. While there, he spent several nights a week volunteering at the Haight Ashbury Free Clinic, one of the first street clinics in America. "I think that was really the first time that I understood that there are things that are happening to our youth that need attention," he said. "I think that's important for many of my generation in moving medicine toward understanding adolescents and the need for our role in helping this population, which in turn helped to make our country and our society better." He laughs, saying he returned from San Francisco thinking he invented the field of adolescent medicine, only to find out that there were formal programs across the country—one of which was at Boston Children's Hospital, where he spent a summer mentored by one of the founders of adolescent medicine, Dr. Robert Masland. His Boston experience solidified for Elster that he wanted to specialize in adolescent medicine.

After medical school, Dr. Elster completed a pediatric residency and chief residency at the University of New Mexico, a time that coincided with the Vietnam War. He enlisted in the military as a member of the Berry Plan, a program that permitted physicians to defer military service until specialty training was complete. This decision proved invaluable to the development of his career.

While rotating in San Francisco during medical school, he met a chief resident, Dr. Joe Sanders. Sanders was not only a leader in adolescent medicine and eventually became executive director of the American Academy of Pediatrics (AAP); he also served as the Consultant to the Surgeon General of the Army. Dr. Sanders helped Dr. Elster receive his military appointment at an Army teaching hospital, Madigan Army Medical Center in Tacoma, Washington, which was in need of an adolescent medicine program. Dr. Elster was asked to develop an adolescent clinic because of his interest and passion in this field. He had no formal training—an incredible experience that "was really training on the job," he said. He spent two and one-half years providing services and teaching residents adolescent medicine. Portending future interest, he also initiated a special multidisciplinary program to care for pregnant teens. For his efforts, Dr. Elster received a Medal of Commendation from the U.S. Army, and a service award from the AAP. During this time, Dr. Elster decided to pursue formal fellowship training and read about the program in Rochester, New York, led by Dr. Elizabeth McAnarney, whom he later met in person at an AAP meeting in Chicago. Finding it to be a great fit, he signed on to come to Rochester when his enlistment and a five-month tour of Europe ended.

Dr. Elster recalls a wonderfully diverse training experience in Rochester. He remembers spending time on the inpatient adolescent unit, at the student health service, and even seeing young musicians at the renowned Eastman School of Music, all experiences that he remembers as extremely valuable. However, he remains most grateful for the opportunity to take courses in grant writing, developing proposals, and handling budgets. "That was incredibly important for the rest of my career in academic medicine," he said. In fact, he says it was through the Rochester fellowship program that he truly learned about academic medicine, something he has devoted his career to ever since. He remains grateful for the role Dr. McAnarney played in introducing him to the Society for Adolescent Medicine (SAM). "She ushered me into the Society, helped me meet people there, and expanded my contacts and my horizons by seeing people around the country who were doing the same thing," he said. He later went on to become the president of the SAM (named Society for Adolescent Health and Medicine [SAHM] in 1997), carrying on a legacy of Rochester alumni and alumnae holding this position. (Five Rochester faculty and/or fellows have served as president thus far.)

In addition to finding his passion in academic medicine while in fellowship, he also developed his primary research interest (young fathers) through working with the unique Rochester Adolescent Maternity Program (RAMP). He remembers sitting in a waiting room one day, talking to a young man whose teenage girlfriend was pregnant. Feeling particularly neglected and left out of the process, this young father-to-be felt there was no place for him, even though he very much wanted a place. This interaction inspired Dr. Elster to look further at this population of young fathers, something he continued to study throughout the rest of his career. His time in Rochester was marked with such pivotal experiences that helped prepare him for the future paths he would take. When he thinks of Rochester Adolescent Medicine, he says he thinks of family. Noting its rich history, beginning with Dr. Stanford B. Friedman and greatly expanded by Dr. McAnarney, he says, "I think there was always a sense of family and connectedness and of value, that we were valued. We valued the people that came before us, and in turn, we valued those of us that came after."

Upon his fellowship graduation, Dr. McAnarney introduced him to the then chair of Pediatrics at the University of Utah, Dr. Lowell Glasgow, who was a graduate of the University of Rochester School of Medicine and Dentistry (URSMD) and had formerly been a member of the pediatric infectious diseases faculty at the University of Rochester. Dr. Glasgow was seeking a faculty candidate to start an Adolescent Medicine program at Utah and hired Dr. Elster to do just that. During his interview, Dr. Elster shared his vision with Dr. Glasgow to develop a teen pregnancy program there, inspired by his work with RAMP in Rochester. In his new program, Dr. Elster would include a special emphasis on engaging young fathers. His colleagues in Utah were very much interested in this concept and welcomed it. Dr. Elster was able to receive State Health Department aid for a nutritionist, nurse practitioner, and midwife, as well as establish a Women, Infants, and Children (WIC) program, ultimately being able to attract almost all pregnant teenagers in the area into this special program at the university. He maintained his goal of introducing special programming targeted toward young fathers through initiatives that involved them in prenatal visits as often as possible, occupational counseling on schooling and careers, as well as coaching programs after delivery.

The International Business Machines (IBM) Corporation was just introducing portable computers, so Dr. Elster and his team were able to develop databases to collect information on the young mothers, fathers, and their babies, and follow them longitudinally for two years. He developed a colleagueship with one of the most prominent developmental psychologists in the country, Dr. Michael Lamb, and together they conducted research and published on young fathers. "Children having children" was an area of emphasis both in medicine and social service and became a focus for both foundations and the federal government. Dr. Elster found himself engaging in national conversations, including appearing on the *Today Show* to discuss his work.

Due to these research successes, he received a five-year Faculty Scholars Development grant from the W.T. Grant Foundation, where he continued his work with young mothers and fathers. Dr. Lamb began working at the National Institutes of Health (NIH) and Dr. Elster briefly joined him for a year to continue their research together. During that year, the AMA created a position in adolescent health to develop programming and recruited Dr. Elster as the first director of the Department of Adolescent Health. "I think that for me philosophically what I was interested in was what kind of shadow did I want to leave," he said, noting that he could leave the largest shadow by working at the national level. "So that really was the impetus for me, and it was where my strength was," he said, which was connecting people, formation of ideas and programmatic development, and "how to connect the dots, especially as you work with adolescents and adolescent health." He spent twenty years at the AMA developing educational programs for physicians and developing policy. Perhaps most notably, through funding from the Centers for Disease Control (CDC), he led the development of a package of preventive services to incorporate into medical care, called the Guidelines for Adolescent Preventive Services (GAPS), still in use today. To promote stronger advocacy, he also formed a National Commission on Adolescent Health, bringing together professionals from over thirty national organizations, something he credits the national platform of the AMA in allowing him to do. "That is the power of bringing a multidisciplinary group together—you can move the world of adolescent healthcare into a different stratosphere," he said.

After spending twenty years at the AMA, he decided it was time to move on, and he pursued a master's degree in jurisprudence with a special focus on maternal-child health at Loyola Law School in Chicago, Illinois. "What it gave me was this Reader's Digest of law that was specifically aimed at children and youth," he said, noting that an inherent aspect of working in adolescent medicine is working closely at the interface of medicine, public health, and the law. These issues include reproductive health, gun rights, consent and confidentiality, mandatory vaccination for school, and more. "It gave me more of a grounding in law, in the constitution, how one works legally with teenagers, and the rights of teenagers," he said. "I think it's really critical for how we develop programs, how we develop structures, and how we develop policies for teenagers—all of that relates to law, and to what their legal and constitutional rights are." At Northwestern University, he developed courses in disease prevention and health promotion, public health law, and global tobacco control and prevention, which he still teaches today through part of the university's MPH program.

Dr. Elster's career has taken several paths, all of which have greatly contributed to improving the health and well-being of adolescents. He remains most proud of the programs he developed—from the Adolescent Medicine program at Madigan Army Medical Center and the teenage pregnancy program at Utah, which is still going strong—to developing GAPS and ultimately helping to bridge medicine and public health while at the AMA and to his current work in developing MPH courses in adolescent health and law. He is also proud that he has been able to influence young people to pursue a career in pediatrics, and specifically adolescent medicine—young minds that will help continue to move the field forward.

As for the future, he says, "I think I would want to look at the role and value of youth in society," explaining that in earlier years, the focus was on the role of health and creating healthy youth. "I don't think we can, nor do I think we should, look at adolescents anymore without looking at social justice and equity," he said, noting that was not necessarily the case during his years of practice. "I would reconvene some of these national commissions to look at the role of adolescent health and social equity. How do we use the power of teenagers? Because I think all of us, myself included, who are in adolescent medicine, have a strong, passionate belief in the goodness and the value of adolescents and what they can add to society."

Dr. Elster's contributions are vast and varied, have certainly cast a big shadow, and have built upon early experiences gained and interests fostered in Rochester. He has witnessed growth and change occur in the field over these past forty years and has contributed greatly on the national stage, significantly influencing how we think about and treat adolescent health across the country.

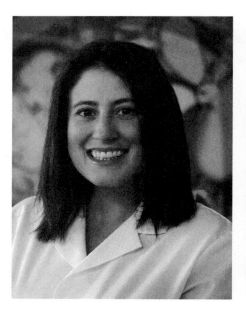

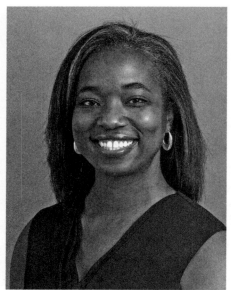

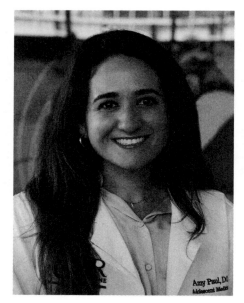

Chapter Seven

FELLOWS (RECENT GRADUATES)

NICOLE CIFRA, MD, MPH, MHPED (2022),
MELISSA A. DUNDAS, MD, FAAP (2021),
AMY Y. PAUL, DO (2023)

The Adolescent Medicine Fellowship program at the University of Rochester (UR) has a long and rich history as one of the earliest programs in the country, serving as the training ground for numerous fellows from diverse backgrounds who have had varied interests. While the program has played an instrumental role in each of their careers, each trainee has also left his/her unique imprint and legacy on the fellowship program. Common themes were uncovered when alumni reminisced on their experiences, including feelings of camaraderie, community, and excellent training. These same themes hold true for the program's current and most recent graduate fellows, Drs. Nicole Cifra (2022), Melissa Dundas (2021), and Amy Paul (2023), who share their thoughts in this piece.

Each of these young physicians was drawn to the UR Adolescent Medicine Fellowship program for similar reasons—the excellent specialized training and a strong sense of community and camaraderie among division members. As soon as Dr. Nicole Cifra was introduced to the field of adolescent medicine as a medical student in Syracuse, she knew she wanted to focus on adolescents who have eating disorders and was drawn to the UR for its national reputation. In fact, she chose Rochester for her pediatric residency training with that fellowship goal in mind. "Being at a place that has a high volume of patients, but also offers a high degree of specialty and expertise drew me here," she said. Dr. Melissa Dundas was drawn to the broad, holistic education provided in Rochester through strong programs in eating disorders, gender health, and gynecology. However, the culture was most important to her. "I wanted to be in an environment that was humane," she said. "Training is so difficult and having finished medical school and residency, I thought this next chapter is more of a choice and so I wanted it to be a place that would allow for me to be human at the same time." This was the environment she experienced in Rochester and that which she described to her former coresident, Dr. Amy Paul, as Dr. Paul applied to fellowship. "[Melissa] told me all about it—how amazing the program was and how amazing the people were," Dr. Paul said. "So, when I came to interview, I just realized that I liked the camaraderie here; I felt like everyone liked each other. I liked the community feeling that was here. That's what drew me to Rochester."

Each of these women found her own niche, which the program supported and helped develop. Dr. Dundas's focus became reproductive and sexual health—"primarily from a reproductive justice health model," she said. "To me, it is super critical because a lot of teenagers of color from low-income areas never have great access to reproductive healthcare. Being able to be an advocate not only in the clinical space, but outside of the hospital, is super important to me and something I'm really passionate about." She is currently an assistant professor of Pediatrics at New York University, focusing on sexual reproductive health, as well as eating disorders and gender health—all three areas in which she believes she received strong training during fellowship. She is helping to build the inpatient eating disorder service and start a gender health program at Bellevue Hospital, which predominantly serves underresourced communities. She says she is thankful for her training in Rochester, attributing it to getting her through a very busy start to her attending career. "I'm the only person in the whole health system who has formal inpatient eating disorder training for medical management and that's because of Rochester," she said, noting that Rochester's is one of the only adolescent medicine fellowship programs in New York State that offers such robust inpatient management of patients who have eating disorders.

Dr. Cifra enjoyed that robust training, never wavering from her passion for eating disorder care. However, she also uncovered new interests, particularly around science communication and media work. During fellowship, she became a spokesperson for the American Academy of Pediatrics (AAP) and became a go-to source for the local media on adolescent health matters, something she plans to continue in her career. She also obtained her Masters in Health Professions Education degree. Following her fellowship graduation in June 2022, she joined the faculty at Children's Hospital of Philadelphia (CHOP) as an assistant professor where she is primarily focusing on eating disorders, as well as some gynecology and primary care. She will be spending some of her inpatient time in a new hospital on a service dedicated to malnutrition and eating disorders and says, "It will be fun and interesting to be a part of something that is new and to see how that develops over time."

Dr. Amy Paul's interest is in LGBTQ+ healthcare and gender affirming care. "My focus is gender medicine and Rochester has a great gender program, but you also get to experience and get an expertise in everything else as well, including reproductive health and eating disorders, which I know will be beneficial for me wherever I go," she said. Dr. Paul is also obtaining her Masters in Health Professions Education, something she said the program has very much supported. She is proud of how much she has learned over the course of two years. Beginning her fellowship with minimal experience with caring for patients who have eating disorders, a need for gender affirming hormone care, or reproductive health including long-acting reversible contraception (LARC), she is now entering her third and final year of fellowship." She reflects, "I came here very fresh, and learning in this short period of time and feeling like an expert in some of these things has been pretty amazing."

When reflecting on Rochester Adolescent Medicine, each had a certain sentiment or word come to mind. "Community," said Dr. Paul. "Everyone supports each other and everyone's main goal is to provide the best affirming care and to be as supportive as we can to our patients. I know if I needed something, I could reach out to at least ten people to help me with any question I have, which I think is great." Dr. Dundas echoed this sentiment: "I think the level of compassion that we shared for each other in this training program actually allows us to be better adolescent medicine doctors," she said. Dr. Cifra is thankful for the training she received and the way it prepared her for her future. "I feel like it has been a really good place for my training interests, and I think I'm definitely well prepared and had a lot of opportunities to develop my interests and plan for next steps," she said. For Dr. Dundas, the word is "grace." "When I think of Rochester and that program, I think of grace—grace with ourselves, grace with patients, grace with the system, and grace with acute and chronic changes. It's just being graceful with our approach and our care at all times," she said.

While still early on in their careers, each has witnessed changes occur in the field—from shifts in popular areas of practice to changes in medical education to new challenges. Dr. Cifra comments on the decline of those interested in eating disorders. "From my perspective, eating disorders has always been a pillar of adolescent health and still is, but I think that more fellows are interested in other things besides eating disorders, so I feel that it's becoming more of a rarity to have that interest," she said. She notes that this shift has become apparent during the COVID-19 pandemic, as eating disorder rates increased, but the population of fellowship graduates interested in that aspect of adolescent medicine has appeared to decrease. She finds this shift to be interesting, but a great opportunity to pursue the work she has always been interested in during a time that it is very much needed.

Dr. Paul has witnessed a positive shift in medical education, even from the time she first began medical school in 2013. "Medical education and providers are becoming more affirming, addressing their implicit biases, and becoming less judgmental," she said. While she says this is a benefit to all patients, it is especially helpful for adolescent patients, who she believes have become more honest and open with themselves and more willing to experiment with who they are. "I think it takes a provider being okay with that and being affirming to that," she said. "I think we're learning that in medical education where in the past we did not, which has been very helpful."

Dr. Dundas has witnessed the field continue to gain more respect. "What I see happening is people starting to respect adolescent medicine more as a specialty and understand that we have such a gift to be able to connect with youth and just get them a little bit over the hump, whereas other individuals may not be able to help get them there," she said. She has also seen new challenges arise. "I do see adolescent mental health issues being the biggest challenge for us to navigate, but it's going to be the biggest success story moving forward in terms of what we're able to do within our sphere of care."

All three of these young physicians completed their training during a notorious time in history that has seen a multiyear global pandemic, social unrest, and a divisive political climate. Dr. Paul noted that we are living in a time when access to care is at risk due to laws being overturned (*Roe v. Wade*) and the stigmatization of certain treatments, including gender-affirming hormones. "I worry for adolescents in the future if we are not able to provide the care they so deserve and require," she said.

They all agreed that advocacy is critical, and it was actually through these challenges that Dr. Dundas recalls one of her fondest memories of her time in Rochester. "What really stood out to me was how the program and division were so ready and willing to adapt and pivot when all the social uprisings were happening in the summer of 2020," she said. She remarks that many youth were experiencing trauma surrounding those events and turned to the adolescent medicine providers to comfort, guide, and take care of them. "It was only possible to do that if we were actually taking an active stance," she said. "So, I really did value that irrespective of the generational differences in the division, we were all able to come together for the common good and truly advocate for our patient population outside of the four walls of the hospital."

All three providers contributed greatly to the Adolescent Medicine Division and fellowship program—from their unique interests and associated clinical and scholarly work to their passions that extended outside of the hospital and into the community to the value they placed on compassionate care toward their patients and each other. As they shared their fond memories of their time in Rochester, several things were evident—the feelings of gratitude for the training they received, pride for the team with whom they worked, and a true passion and commitment to adolescent health.

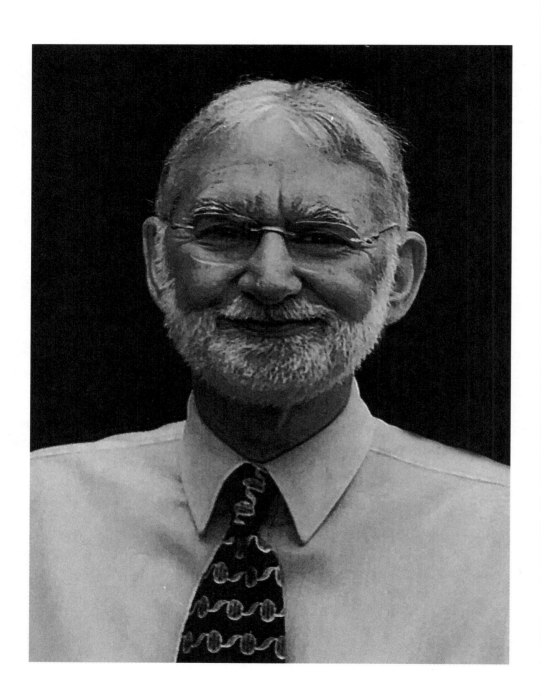

Chapter Eight

MAURY FRIEMAN, EdD, MSW, MSc

Maury Frieman grew up in Baltimore, Maryland, the youngest of three siblings. His childhood and adolescence were significantly affected by his father's chronic illness and death when Maury was only seventeen years old. He had to become an advocate for his father during his hospitalizations, and became comfortable in the hospital environment, an experience that would serve him in his later professional life. It helped him to understand the emotional impact on families when a member of the family is hospitalized. At the same time, he learned very early to advocate for himself. In addition, he was close with his older brother, a professor of early childhood education, who was his major support. He credits his brother with helping him develop resilience and with building his self-esteem and eventually steering him toward a career working with children and adolescents.

Frieman attended the University of Maryland, Baltimore County (UMBC). He was able to develop his own degree program, with the support of Dr. Trudy Hamby. The degree was a combination of an early childhood education program that was based on humanistic psychology theory and clinical social work, and was directed by Dr. Hamby. His goal was to gain the knowledge and competency of a play therapist for hospitalized children. During an early childhood internship in the Pediatrics Department at Sinai Hospital, Baltimore, his supervisor went out on leave and he was asked to take her place for four months, an invaluable experience.

Following graduation, Frieman took a position as a play therapist/child life worker on the Adolescent Unit in the Department of Pediatrics at the University of Maryland Medical Center. This unit was directed by Dr. Felix Heald. It was during this time that Dr. Stanford Friedman moved from Rochester to Maryland to begin the Behavioral Pediatrics program there. It was an environment where Frieman could take the initiative to attend conferences and learn from residents and staff trained in behavioral medicine, with a focus on the whole child. A workshop by Dr. Elizabeth Kubler-Ross led to the development of his expertise in addressing the clinical issues of death and dying with pediatric patients and their families.

Maury worked closely with Marilyn Aten, RN, MS, PhD, who left the University of Maryland Medical Center to join the nursing faculty at the University of Rochester's Strong Memorial Hospital (SMH). She strongly encouraged Maury to apply for the position of adolescent child life worker at Rochester, which he did. Thus, in 1975, he moved to Rochester and began working as a child life worker at SMH on the Adolescent Unit (unit 4-1400). It was here that he defined his career path. He credits his experiences working as part of the inpatient adolescent medicine team with inspiring and shaping much of his future career as a social worker and therapist. The unit was led by Dr. Elizabeth McAnarney, and utilized a team approach to meet the patients' psychosocial and emotional needs while hospitalized for medical and surgical treatment. Maury described his role on the adolescent unit as working with adolescents throughout the course of their hospitalization, using play therapy and counseling, while collaborating with the medical and social work staff. Maury worked with adolescents challenged by brief, prolonged, or recurrent hospitalization due to medical and surgical concerns or treatment for eating disorders. In particular, he gained experience working with terminally ill patients and their families. This became a significant part of his later clinical practice. The goal of the team was to help the hospitalized adolescent cope with the multiple issues surrounding their hospitalization and medical concerns, in order to reduce the stress of hospitalization and separation from their normal environment, and to help patients feel like "kids" and not just a medical diagnosis. Team meetings were focused on the whole child. In contrast to the traditional medical model, the contribution of every team member, irrespective of their professional degree, was encouraged, valued and respected by Dr. McAnarney. This inclusiveness and respect, as well as the many clinical lessons provided by Dr. McAnarney, became the model for Dr. Frieman's approach to working with patients, families, and colleagues in his professional practice throughout his career. Further, through working with adolescent medicine nursing staff, medical residents, and attendings, as well as with prominent psychiatrist Dr. Christopher Hodgman and attending classes led by Dr. George Engel, creator of the biopsychosocial model, he broadened and deepened his professional skills. "Of all my professional positions I've held, none has ever come close to this kind of formative environment, and never will," he said.

While at Rochester, Maury was encouraged and supported when he decided to continue his education in order to add to his knowledge base and professional skills. He pursued an MSc in Community Services, the focus of which was to work with people in the context of their environment to build support, while working full time on the adolescent unit. In Rochester, he also met and married Dr. Alyne Ricker, who was a pediatric resident at SMH, and in1980, they moved to Calgary, Alberta, Canada, for Alyne's first pediatric endocrinology fellowship year. Maury was able to obtain a position as mental health clinician on the Adolescent Psychiatry Unit at Foothills Hospital. A year later, Maury continued his professional development when enrolling in a MSW degree in a psychoanalytically based program at Smith College School for social work. His one-year internship was at Boston Children's Hospital Psychosomatic Unit. There, when assigned to treat individual patients and families, he was challenged by length of stay limitations imposed by insurance. Through these limitations, he had to learn to develop trust quickly in order to provide appropriate therapy and support. At Children's he was fortunate to be mentored by Drs. Gordon Harper and T. Berry Brazelton, experts in the fields of child psychiatry and pediatrics.

In subsequent years, Maury was a clinician in community mental health, and was a social worker in a pediatric Intensive Care Unit (ICU) at Rhode Island Hospital. Following his wife's career opportunity in North Carolina, he found a position as social work supervisor in the Departments of Psychiatry and Rehabilitation at East Carolina University School of Medicine.

Additionally, he was a therapist in an inpatient psychiatry unit serving adults and adolescents, followed by being a therapist in a private psychiatric hospital for children and adolescents, and subsequently he went into private practice. While in North Carolina, he aspired to do something more for children and adolescents in the community, and cofounded a therapeutic horseback-riding program for emotionally and physically challenged children. Back in Massachusetts, he also served as mental health consultant and therapist at a camp for children who had diabetes.

During these years, he experienced the challenges of managed care that placed limitations on ambulatory treatment of children and families. He began seeking alternative ways to use his experience and clinical strengths, and pursued a position in the schools. In school, he was able to work with children and families, consult with teachers, and be an active presence in the community. He could work with children across the developmental spectrum. As he was often one of the first to be called in crises that seriously affected students, such as death of a family member or a student, he has helped families through their most vulnerable heartbreaking times and has created lifelong bonds.

To expand his knowledge in this new environment and support his work with students he attended the University of Massachusetts, Lowell, and earned his EdD focused on leadership in schools. This was a most rewarding time professionally. He received his degree in the same year in which his daughter earned her Bachelor of Arts from Yale University and was named a Rhodes Scholar.

In describing this winding career path that centered on helping children and adolescents, there are common themes. These are modeled on Dr. Frieman's experiences and knowledge learned when working as part of the Adolescent Medicine team in Rochester. He continued to broaden and deepen his professional expertise through education and training and sought out expert (and willing) mentors like Dr. McAnarney, and others mentioned above, who taught him to listen to and to treat his patients with respect and dignity. "My time in Rochester clearly shaped my career, and shaped my hunger to learn as much as I can as well as the way I went about dealing with people professionally my whole life."

Throughout his career, Dr. Frieman has counseled, comforted, advocated for, supported, and cared for countless people, playing an instrumental role in the lives of these children, adolescents, patients, students, and families. It is a calling and gift to be able to walk alongside others in times of difficulty and suffering—a gift that he surely has and so selflessly shares.

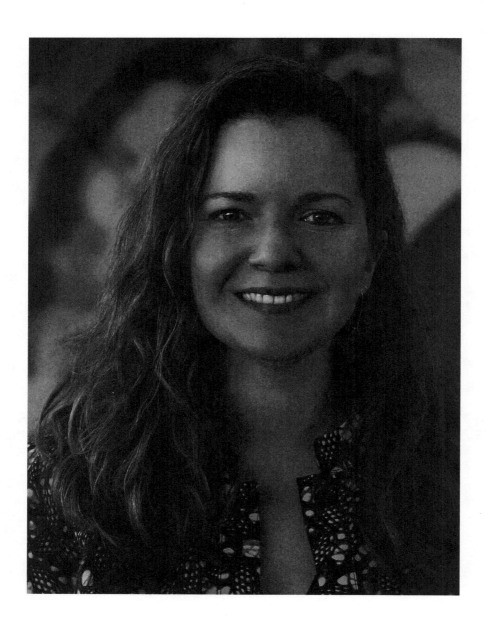

Chapter Nine

KATHERINE BLUMOFF GREENBERG, MD

Katherine "Kate" Greenberg has been a strong advocate for marginalized persons for as long as she can remember. A 2007 medical graduate of the University of Rochester School of Medicine and Dentistry (URSMD) and a 2014 graduate of the University of Rochester Adolescent Medicine Fellowship program, she remains in Rochester as a valued faculty member. She is currently an associate professor of Pediatrics (Adolescent Medicine) and Obstetrics and Gynecology (General Gynecology) and vice chair for Diversity and Cultural Development for the Department of Pediatrics, leading the way in gender health and diversity, equity, and inclusion.

Greenberg married into a long line of Greenberg physicians, but she was the first person in her family-of-origin to pursue medicine. Looking back, she said she had really been training for a career in adolescent medicine for much of her life. In high school, she was an unofficial peer-counselor for her friends, helping them through various adolescent issues. When she entered Johns Hopkins University for her undergraduate education, she became involved with their formal peer-counseling program, ultimately serving as a leader directing the training program for new counselors. In this role, she ran several positive youth development sexual health sessions with local students in high schools in Baltimore, facilitating conversations about relationships and reproductive health choices.

When she started college, she became a public health major and aspired to be an Epidemiology Intelligence Service (EIS) Officer. She laughs, saying that after reading *The Hot Zone* she thought that being a "disease detective" was in her future. "I was really interested in global health, but it became clear to me that I wanted to be able to provide health care and contribute to community health," she said. That interest led her to study abroad her junior year in Nairobi, Kenya—an experience that solidified her decision to become a physician when she saw patients who were experiencing unmet medical needs that she might address. By pursuing medicine, "I knew that I could contribute to public policy and advocacy, but I also knew that I would have some tangible skills that I could really take with me into various settings," she said. Her international work has continued with trips to Honduras, Poland, and Haiti following the earthquake, where one of her proudest achievements remains placing an IV in a severely dehydrated three-year-old who was in an informal tent camp. She used a headlamp and moderated by hand the number of drips per second going into the IV bag. She successfully rehydrated the child, who needed IV fluids that were not available anywhere else in Port-au-Prince.

Her interest in LGBTQ+ health, now a major focus of her career, also developed early on. Though she says it sounds stereotypical, she attended a performing arts high school and had peers who identified as part of the LGBTQ+ community. In fact, she remembers her first transgender peer when she was just fourteen, a rarity in 1994. Through her peer counseling experiences in college, she did a great deal of work with LGBTQ+ community members, and during the year following college as she applied for medical school, she worked with a lesbian health project in Buffalo, New York. Through this experience, she had the opportunity to attend the National Lesbian Health Conference and to work with local LGBTQ+ youth groups, to whom she had to navigate "coming out" as a straight woman. "I had a year of experiencing as much as a straight, cis person can, an empathy-building experience around living with sexuality that is different from what other people assume about you," she said.

Greenberg chose to attend the University of Rochester School of Medicine and Dentistry (URSMD) for her medical education in large part because of the collaborative learning environment and the biopsychosocial model developed there in 1977, still a major theme in the university's medical school. "The biopsychosocial model really spoke to my need for that public health perspective," she said. "That is, we're not looking at individual health, but we're really looking at each individual as part of a much larger biopsychosocial sphere." It was during medical school in Rochester that she learned about adolescent medicine and that her experiences up to this point were perfectly aligned with a career in that field. She also knew she was passionate about and committed to sexual and reproductive freedom and came into medical school knowing she wanted to be able to provide the full spectrum of women's healthcare. She considered a residency in obstetrics and gynecology (OBGYN) but, knowing that she ultimately wanted to pursue adolescent medicine, she chose an internship in family medicine before completing a residency in pediatrics at Rainbow Babies and Children's Hospital in Cleveland, Ohio.

When pursuing fellowship programs, she was drawn back to the biopsychosocial atmosphere at Rochester. It was also important to her to find a program that would help foster opportunities for reproductive health training. Dr. Susan "Shellie" Yussman, Rochester's fellowship program director, was committed to allowing trainees to pursue individualized interests and facilitating the necessary opportunities. Dr. Greenberg was also familiar with Dr. Rachael Phelps, the medical director at Planned Parenthood, and knew she could receive training in procedural abortion as an adolescent medicine fellow. Her fellowship also enabled training in intrauterine device (IUD) and NEXPLANON insertion. These experiences allowed her to develop and then eventually bring to the faculty group a unique sexual and reproductive health expertise, ultimately enabling her to help broaden the program's reproductive health services. Rochester's program also gave her the incredible opportunity to learn from Dr. Elizabeth McAnarney, whom she refers to as one of the "matriarchs of the field of adolescent medicine," something for which she is extremely grateful.

During Dr. Greenberg's second year of fellowship, Dr. Mandy Coles relocated to Boston, Massachusetts; Dr. Coles led the division's nascent gender health initiatives, and had a cohort of about 15–20 patients who were transgender. Upon Dr. Coles' departure, Dr. Yussman was supportive of Dr. Greenberg taking over this panel of patients under the preceptorship of faculty from pediatric and adult endocrinology. When Dr. Greenberg decided to stay in

Rochester upon her graduation, she officially assumed leadership for this gender health program, formalized it through marketing and outreach initiatives, and witnessed its tremendous growth. As the largest program in Central and Western New York, Gender Health Services at Golisano Children's Hospital served nearly 500 unique patients and families in 2020. Dr. Greenberg is extremely proud of this expansion and attributes it greatly to the "flexibility and 'we can make that work' attitude of the division," she says. "Really I'm most proud of helping us become one of the centers that's on the crest of the wave of a national movement in terms of caring for transgender youth," she said. She notes that the American Academy of Pediatrics (AAP) developed a position statement in support of affirming care for transgender youth in 2018, but Rochester has been providing such care since 2012 and has garnered national attention. "I've been doing this now for eight years and so I have a lot of patients who came as early teens who are now young adults living their best lives. That is just incredibly gratifying," she said. It has also offered a remarkable training experience for fellows who all spend a significant amount of time in gender health clinic with Dr. Greenberg and graduate fully capable of caring for gender diverse youth.

In 2018, the chair of the Department of Pediatrics, Dr. Patrick Brophy, named Dr. Greenberg the vice chair for Diversity and Cultural Development, which she believes was sponsored by Dr. McAnarney in recognition of her advocacy efforts in gender and sexual and reproductive health. She is proud of the institution for making this a priority and for being at the forefront of focusing on inclusion. She was a member of the steering committee for a new Association of American Medical Colleges (AAMC) Assessment for Inclusive Climate and presented nationally on Rochester's initiatives. When the COVID-19 pandemic hit in 2020, followed by a remarkable increase in awareness of racial inequities, she said the university was extremely well-positioned to address inclusivity and health equity. "I'm really proud of our leadership for having made this a priority even before national momentum," she said, "because it gave us a really nice ability to take advantage of that momentum and move forward." She believes her background in adolescent medicine has helped her greatly in this role. "We appreciate the opportunity to have hard conversations to facilitate self-discovery and development," she said. "I think of us fundamentally as developmental people trying to help shape the life-course of young people so that they can be healthy and successful. And I think we are not afraid of challenging issues and are able to engage in hard questions and push the limits a little bit, which is a skill set that naturally lends itself to advocacy and then to having those hard conversations and perspective."

She believes this advocacy is the future of the field of adolescent medicine, as well. "Nationally, we're moving in the direction of social justice, and I hope that we are carving out a breadth of roles for ourselves as adolescent health specialists," she said. She served as the 2020–2021 Education Committee Chair for the Society for Adolescent Health and Medicine (SAHM). They created a webinar series called "Adolescent Medicine as a Tool for Social Justice," which reflects the multiple ways in which adolescent medicine providers can advocate and discuss social justice and antiracism. She hopes that as a field adolescent medicine can work within academic medical centers to value diversity, equity, and inclusion—something in which she has faith given the continuous transformation of the field. "I think the specialty is so young and we've come so far," she said, acknowledging the tremendous evolution that has occurred in the past fifty years, let alone in just the eight years that she has been out of fellowship. From Dr. McAnarney's seminal work demonstrating that with developmentally directed care to pregnant adolescents, both mothers and infants can have optimal outcomes, to now talking about reproductive justice and antiracism for adolescents, she finds it remarkable just how dramatically the field has evolved. She is also proud of the way it has influenced pediatrics. "The degree to which our pediatric residency program focuses on contraception as an essential health service, on adolescent care and gender health care as essential to our care of children, is huge," she said. Additionally, in 2020 she became the director of the Susan B. Anthony and Frederick Douglass Scholars Program for the Department of Pediatrics. This novel pediatric educational program aims to provide pediatricians with competence in research, advocacy, medical education, or an individualized skill set in understanding health inequity, with focuses on racial and gender equity.

In each of Dr. Greenberg's contributions to the Division of Adolescent Medicine, Department of Pediatrics, and field as a whole, innovation is an apparent common thread. "I think that innovative spirit is part of the legacy here," she said. "I think a fundamental strength of the program is openness and the ability to grow. I've had interests that were not part of what we had been doing but could be a part of the future, and people have really nurtured that." She credits the leadership for giving her that freedom and permission to bring new foci to the program. "I'm allowed to be innovative and am encouraged and nurtured in creating new service lines and adding to our education, our patient care, and our research, which is something that's really valued," she said.

Dr. Greenberg's unique expertise in sexual, reproductive and gender health, with her special innovative spirit, advocacy efforts, and encouragement for change, have all contributed to Rochester's program and the field of adolescent medicine in significant ways and is improving care for adolescents globally. She is emerging as a major innovator and creative academician in adolescent medicine who brings her talent and continual intellectual growth to her patients, families, and colleagues.

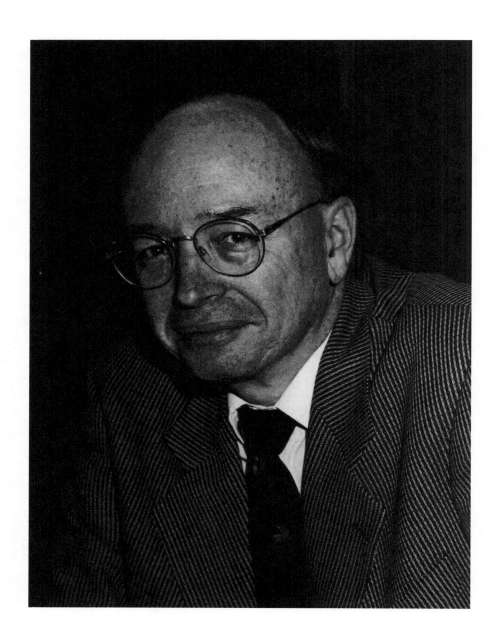

Chapter Ten

Donald E. Greydanus, MD, Dr. HC (Athens)

Donald E. Greydanus has spent his career caring for adolescents, developing and leading programs to improve training and care, and promoting the field of adolescent medicine to international audiences. An avid reader and writer, he finds many parallels in his life to the stories written by Charles Dickens. Dickens once said, "The most important thing in life is to stop saying 'I wish' and start saying 'I will,'" which is something Dr. Greydanus has truly embodied. "I have always followed the Charles Dickens philosophy of 'Don't say you want to do something, go try it'—get out there and see what life opens up," he said. Throughout his forty-plus-year career, life has opened many opportunities for him and one for which he is extremely grateful is his first faculty position as an assistant professor of Pediatrics in the Division of Adolescent Medicine at the University of Rochester from 1978 to 1983. He remembers those years fondly as an integral chapter of his own story and is grateful for the impact it had on the rest of his career.

Greydanus was born in Paterson, New Jersey. His father was an engineer and his mother was a nurse who encouraged him from a young age to consider a career in medicine. While his childhood dreams consisted of becoming a concert pianist at Carnegie Hall or a replacement for Mickey Mantle on the New York Yankees, he laughs, saying he wasn't quite good enough for either, so he decided to try medicine. He attended Calvin College in Grand Rapids, Michigan, for his undergraduate education and returned to New Jersey for medical school in Newark at what is now Rutgers Medical School.

He remarks how certain instances can occur on any given day that greatly impact one's life, and one such occasion for him was during his surgery clerkship as a third-year medical student when one of his preceptors suggested he consider training at Mayo Clinic in Rochester, Minnesota. Taking this professor's advice, he interviewed there for his pediatric residency, fell in love with their philosophy and program, and moved to what would become his "first Rochester."

While at Mayo Clinic, two more significant life events occurred: he met his future wife, Kathy and was invited by President Richard Nixon to go to Vietnam as a General Medical Officer. While he could have deferred his enlistment, he said he had relatives who fought and died in World War II and believed it was his duty and call to serve. He looks back on it as an amazing adventure, and while it was certainly a very difficult time, it was also a time that inspired his interest in adolescent medicine. "As I was contemplating what I wanted to do, one of the things that fascinated me about my time in the Vietnam War zone was how older teenagers and young adults handled stress," he said. "I found that absolutely fascinating—how some did well, some did not, and how do you help them?" He returned to Rochester, Minnesota, and married, finished his residency at Mayo, and then headed back East to New York for a fellowship in Adolescent and Young Adult Medicine at New York University's Bellevue Hospital, training under Dr. Adele Dellenbaugh Hofmann (a founder of adolescent medicine and a graduate of the University of Rochester School of Medicine and Dentistry).

As the end of his fellowship neared, another pivotal life moment occurred for him when Dr. Hofmann suggested he consider going to Rochester, New York, to work with Dr. Elizabeth McAnarney. He had aspirations that were rooted in a bit more wanderlust, however, as he dreamed of going to the Netherlands to spend time in the Endocrine Department at Rotterdam Children's Hospital—learning about endocrinology, as well as the Dutch and Frisian languages of his family's heritage. However, having started his family while in Minnesota and with plans to grow his family, he decided to visit Rochester, where he was immediately drawn to the program and to Dr. McAnarney's strong leadership. Thus, in what he refers to as his own "Tale of Two Cities" (or Tale of Two Rochesters in his case), he soon signed onto moving to his "second Rochester." He found himself impressed by its strong legacy in research and academics, noting that he has yet to see another place that has such a "wonderful combination of excellent clinical care with the emphasis on education and research. It was a wonderful trio," he said. "I thought I was in heaven at the time with the three things I loved to do the most."

While at the University of Rochester, Dr. Greydanus served as the director of the adolescent medicine clinic, learning how to integrate adolescent medicine with other subspecialties such as endocrinology, gynecology, and psychiatry, as well as spent time on the inpatient unit. He was introduced to an aspect of the field that he had not fully experienced previously—the care of patients who had eating disorders—something for which Rochester's program was well known, and an experience he later applied throughout his career. "In life you're always learning, everywhere you go," he said. He was also charged by the then-chair of Pediatrics, Dr. David H. Smith, to teach the pediatric residents about adolescent gynecology, one of his primary clinical and scholarly interests.

His research interests were fostered, as he worked on a number of projects. "I have this condition called *cacoëthes scribendi*—an incurable itch to write," he said. It has become a major outlet in his career, allowing him to author and edit over fifty books with collaborators around the world. One of his proudest contributions is coauthoring and coediting several editions of the textbook *Adolescent Medicine* with Dr. Hofmann, along with the work he continues to publish today. While his research interests have primarily focused on sexual and reproductive health, over the years this interest has expanded to delving into individual organ systems and disease processes and their relation to adolescent health on both a physiological and psychological/emotional basis. His time spent in Vietnam and his curiosity surrounding how adolescents and young adults coped served as a major inspiration for including the emotional piece. His Vietnam experience also influenced his major research interest during his time in Rochester, which was that of contraception, as he found he was much more interested in preventing (an injury during the war, or a medical condition in practice), rather than treating. This interest in prevention worked in great parallel with Dr. McAnarney's interest and leadership in adolescent pregnancy; they had a great collaboration through the esteemed Rochester Adolescent Maternity Program (RAMP).

Along with the remarkable clinical, educational, and scholarly experiences he gained during his University of Rochester faculty tenure, some of his fondest memories remain the people with whom he worked, as he said he found himself meeting one fascinating individual after another. "I think of all the wonderful people that I met—how kind, nice, and reaffirming they were, how interested they were in helping me, this middle-class guy from Paterson, New Jersey, promote what I was doing," he said. He was struck by the willingness of those around him to share—both ideas and learning experiences—something he said does not occur everywhere. "I just think of it as a little bit of a fairy tale."

In 1983, he experienced yet another pivotal moment in his career when he was offered the opportunity to develop an Adolescent Medicine program at Blank Children's Hospital in Des Moines, Iowa. Eager to implement what he had learned from Drs. Hofmann and McAnarney and the influential programs each built, he took the "go and do it" Charles Dickens approach and began writing the next chapter of his story in Des Moines. He started by developing an ambulatory clinic, which ultimately grew into a fourteen-bed inpatient unit within the children's hospital consisting of both day treatment and ambulatory components for teenagers throughout the state of Iowa who were struggling with anxiety, depression, eating disorders, substance abuse, and everything in the behavioral medicine arena except for schizophrenia, other psychoses, and violence. Dr. Greydanus served as medical director for several years while also holding a faculty appointment at the University of Iowa where he was able to collaborate and implement adolescent education there, as well. During this time, he was also asked to be the associate program director of the pediatric residency program at the Blank Children's Hospital and found himself becoming immersed in the world of the Accreditation Council for Graduate Medical Education (ACGME) during a time when requirements were increasing (including increasing subspecialty exposure and scholarly activity). When the director left, Dr. Greydanus assumed the role of chair and program director for several years.

In 1990, he received another remarkable opportunity. The pediatric residency program in Kalamazoo, Michigan, had struggled to adhere to the recent ACGME changes and was losing its accreditation. Dr. Greydanus helped turn the program around. Something he said he learned from Drs. McAnarney and Hofmann and his mentors at Mayo was "always try to do some good for people and help out children." He saw a real opportunity to help improve training, and in turn, improve the health care of children in the greater community. He was able to use the ACGME requirements to bring subspecialists into the Kalamazoo area—colleagues in pediatric endocrinology gastroenterology, nephrology, behavioral pediatrics, and of course adolescent medicine. As he recruited these subspecialists, he says he drew upon a key interpersonal trait he learned from Dr. McAnarney: "being kind to people." In an amazing win-win situation, within three years the residency program improved, as did the care of area children and families who no longer had to travel over 100 miles away to see a subspecialist, but had incredible offerings in their own community. Now over thirty years later, the residency program remains continuously reaccredited and the subspecialist pool remains broad and strong.

In 2010, the president of Western Michigan University in Kalamazoo developed a medical school at the university and the founding dean named Dr. Greydanus the founding chair of the Department of Pediatrics. Greydanus had the great honor of naming the department and aptly chose the Department of Pediatric *and* Adolescent Medicine at Western Michigan University Homer Stryker M.D. School of Medicine. He served as founding chair and the Adolescent Medicine Fellowship program director for several years, and continues part-time in a research capacity today.

Throughout the years, Dr. Greydanus has had the opportunity to chase that wanderlust that grabbed hold of him early on, as he travels internationally to introduce and promote the field of adolescent medicine. It was actually during his time in Rochester, New York, that he was given the opportunity to deliver his first international lecture in 1979. "A lot of things I picked up were stimulated by Rochester and Lissa and have continued to this day," he said. "I'm very grateful for my time there." He has since had the opportunity to travel to places he originally visited when stationed in Vietnam, a full-circle moment for him, in addition to cities throughout Europe and Asia. He has made connections with colleagues around the world, and in 2010, received an honorary doctorate degree from the University of Athens School of Medicine in Greece.

Dr. Greydanus has accomplished much in his career. He says above all, he is most proud of his family, which consists of his wife (Kathy), four daughters (Marissa, Elizabeth, Suzanne, and Megan), and now thirteen grandchildren (four granddaughters and nine grandsons)—"a total and complete joy." He has taken something he learned in Rochester, "Try to make a difference wherever you can be," and has applied that to his career—from writing books and articles, which he said is his way of thanking his mentors, to promoting the field and building collaborations throughout the world. "The joy of adolescent and young adult medicine," he says, "is that you work as a team and you produce a product by working together, not alone." As for the future of the field, he believes there is still a ways to go in continuing to promote the subspecialty, which will require even more adolescent medicine providers to become senior leaders in medical schools, along with the continued strong and important work of the Society for Adolescent Health and Medicine (SAHM). He views the Rochester program as a national leader and remains proud of the strong presence adolescent medicine has historically had and continues to have on the institution, the community, and the field as a whole.

Dr. Greydanus has spent over forty years improving the health of adolescents. He has developed multiple programs and initiatives that have enhanced clinical care, as well as training and education for the next generation, and has extensively published on broad matters applying to adolescent health while promoting the field on national and international stages. In 2017, he was named a distinguished Mayo Clinic alumnus—an honor he says was made possible by his time with Lissa McAnarney in Rochester, New York. Indeed, a true tale of two cities for Don Greydanus! He has truly followed the Charles Dickens approach of not just wishing, but making it happen—and in turn, has written an impressive life story that contributes greatly to the care of adolescents throughout the world.

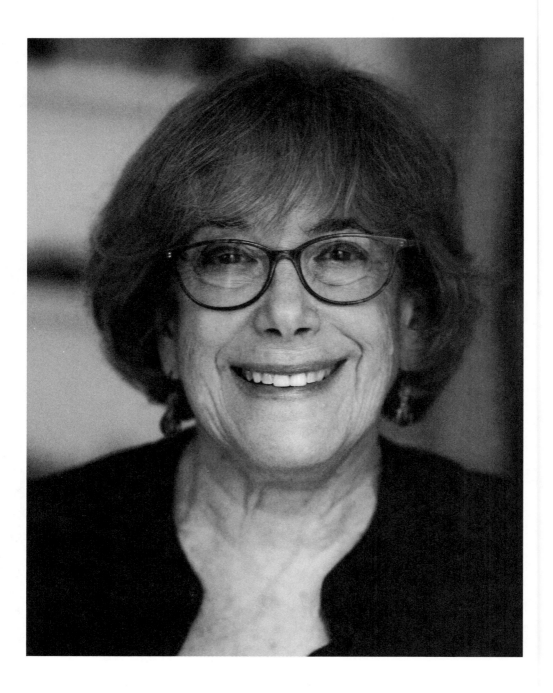

Chapter Eleven

Lisa B. Handwerker, MD, FAAP

Lisa Handwerker has spent her entire career advocating for adolescents and championing adolescent health issues, creating influential change in the communities she has served. Rochester is one such community that truly benefited from her work. She is a 1981 graduate of the General Academic Pediatrics/Adolescent Medicine Fellowship program and served as a valued faculty member for twenty-six years. Her leadership has spanned the local, state and national levels, as she has held roles within the American Academy of Pediatrics (AAP), served as medical director for a major not-for-profit multidisciplinary social service and antipoverty agency, and served as a strong advocate for school-based health centers (SBHCs) across New York State.

Handwerker grew up in the Bronx, New York, until she was six years old, when her family moved to a suburb just outside of New York City. Her grandparents were immigrants from Eastern Europe and her parents grew up in poverty. Education was always an important part of her childhood, but she did not always envision medicine as her career. She attended Case Western Reserve University, planning to major in anthropology before changing her major to special education. She became fascinated with science and medicine after taking a biology course and credits her change in career direction to her professor. Handwerker received her medical degree from Loyola University with her goal to become a pediatrician. In fact, she remembers writing a paper during college in which she expressed the desire to go into adolescent medicine. She said at that time, she was not even sure if it was a specialty, but she was drawn to the age group, and even though she loved her pediatrician, as a teenager she did not like sitting in a waiting room with babies and children. Thus was born Dr. Handwerker's goal of providing medical care for teenagers predominantly.

After completing her pediatrics residency at Long Island Jewish-Hillside Medical Center, Dr. Handwerker was accepted for fellowship training at the University of Rochester. At the time, it was a combined General Academic Pediatrics and Adolescent Medicine program run jointly by Dr. Robert Hoekelman and Dr. Elizabeth McAnarney, leaders who both chaired the Pediatric Department in Rochester. "It was a unique program because they were training you to be an academician and that was exciting to me," she said, noting that she learned skills and had opportunities she would otherwise have had to seek on her own. "It was an opportunity to train to be a leader in the field." She remembers her fellowship as a combination of clinical and scholarly work with the latter consisting of taking courses in medical writing, grant application, and basic accounting principles to aid in budget planning. Dr. Handwerker recalls that her clinical training was phenomenal, practicing in the ambulatory and inpatient settings, consulting for behavioral and medical reasons, and receiving a strong foundation in caring for patients who had eating disorders. However, the experience that she was most passionate about, and upon which she built her career, was her weekly clinic session at Threshold, a drop-in health center for teens. "That's really what I wanted to do with my life," she said.

Threshold was a freestanding, not-for-profit center that provided comprehensive programming in education, vocation, recreation, and medical and behavioral health for adolescents. Upon graduation from her fellowship, Dr. Handwerker became the center's medical director, a role she held for twenty-four years. She was involved with grant writing and was responsible for multiple externally funded programs through the center, and always taught medical and nursing students, residents, and fellows who rotated through the clinic. The programming at Threshold was wide and varied, including a General Education Development (GED) program, a job placement program, substance abuse prevention through providing alternative recreational activities, mental health counseling, and medical services. "It was a really nice place to provide comprehensive care to adolescents combining social determinants of health and medical care," she said. Threshold focused on accessibility to services for patients—not requiring parental permission, eliminating financial barriers, and operating on a time schedule that worked for adolescents, seeing them both by appointment and on a walk-in basis. In addition, Threshold was notably one of the very first SBHCs in the state of New York, and oversaw multiple SBHCs throughout the city of Rochester. She is proud of the impact and change in these centers through advocacy—she cites one example of providing contraception at the SBHCs, a unique offering at the time that required working through the school board and superintendent. She has continued advocating for SBHCs throughout her career, which has culminated in efforts that are greatly responsible for the state legislature's stabilization of SBHC funding in New York State.

In 2004, Dr. Handwerker was recruited to New York City to become the medical director and chief medical officer for Children's Aid, one of the largest multidisciplinary social service agencies in the country. When she joined the organization, originally founded in 1850, it was serving approximately 70,000 families a year through a variety of different disciplines and programs in forty-two centers throughout New York City. Seven of these were health centers, with just half serving an adolescent population. Right before Dr. Handwerker joined, the organization received a Title X grant for family planning. "This was so exciting to me because I had a tremendous amount of experience in implementing those programs from my work at Threshold," she said. However, she notes that while her job at Children's Aid was similar to her work at Threshold, there was a major added component of working with the child welfare system, as the health centers served as primary care providers to 1,500 patients a year who were in foster care. The age range was also wider, as they cared for children from birth to twenty-two years. "It was a steep learning curve for me, not only managing the workings of this huge agency of which I became one of the leaders, but also providing direct patient care and additionally supervising staff who were providers of children from birth on, and learning the entire foster care system in New York City," she said.

However, Handwerker met these challenges and dove right in, leveraging the Title X grant funds to start multiple adolescent reproductive health programs, ultimately expanding these services to adolescents in the Bronx, Manhattan, and Staten Island. This included seeking cooperation from the other pediatrician providers, none of whom was an adolescent specialist and, thus, had to learn how to do contraceptive and sexually transmitted infection (STI) care and treatment. She said it was important to "understand the difference between providing general primary care and to really work to embed good adolescent health care into primary care." As such, they were the first practice site in New York State to train pediatricians and pediatric nurse practitioners to provide long-acting reversible contraceptives (LARC), and even had pediatricians on staff to insert intrauterine devices (IUDs). Under Dr. Handwerker's leadership, Children's Aid has become a leader in New York State that provides adolescent health care to teens and young adults. It is now regarded as a leading program by the New York State and New York City Departments of Health.

Utilizing her experience and passion for school-based health, Dr. Handwerker led Children's Aid to have an influence on health education services in community agencies and schools throughout New York City. Under her leadership, Children's Aid created a model program whereby a health educator would go into middle and high school classrooms to teach and provide office hours on-site in the school where adolescents could drop by to ask questions, as well as provide appointments at the Children's Aid health centers. Furthermore, they were running comprehensive adolescent pregnancy prevention programming in approximately fifteen schools in New York City, with their SBHC in Staten Island to become the first Staten Island program to provide IUDs on-site in a high school setting. Realizing the positive impact these varied programs were having, the New York City Department of Health asked permission to use their model as a basis for a citywide program, for which they received federal funds and subsequently significantly reduced the teen pregnancy rate in New York City by providing access to medical contraception services for teens.

Dr. Handwerker takes pride in her work with Children's Aid—truly embedding quality adolescent healthcare into general pediatric practice that serves under-resourced communities. Dr. Handwerker believes she has used the educational and professional experiences she received in Rochester to influence health initiatives. "It's what I've learned in my fellowship about being a leader that has enabled me to establish relationships, to be able to plan, to advocate, and to think," she said. The initiatives that Dr. Handwerker has led include serving as the only pediatrician on a New York City Department of Health and Mental Hygiene working group tasked with improving the quality of care for adolescents in the city; advocating at the local, state, and federal level for family planning; and as previously mentioned, advocating for SBHCs, which involved discussions with the governor and state legislature, resulting in securing stable state funding. She also served as the president of her chapter of the AAP and is proud of the focus she put on equity and inclusion, expanding their membership and leadership to now representing 1,800 pediatricians in New York City and its surrounding northern counties. "It has been a tremendously rewarding experience for me," she said. "I know for those pediatricians, they feel at home, they feel comfortable now and want to do the work that needs to be done on behalf of children and pediatricians in our region."

Throughout her career, Dr. Handwerker has witnessed the field of adolescent medicine expand and she believes teenagers' health is improving as a result. "I think that the training programs are really making sure that pediatricians and family medicine residents receive a broad exposure to adolescent health," she said, which includes increased training in reproductive and mental health issues. Thus, many are "showing interest in continuing to serve adolescents as they move into whatever practice specialty they are in," she said. Handwerker herself continues to learn and grow in her practice. After retiring from her full-time position at Children's Aid in December 2020, she is expanding her skillset by taking part in a national training program to learn to perform abortions, where she will then be placed in under-resourced communities throughout the United States to fill in for providers as needed. She credits her background in adolescent medicine and reproductive health for enabling her to take this next step in her career.

Dr. Handwerker's leadership and advocacy efforts have pushed the boundaries of the field and have resulted in significant progress and change for communities at the local, state, and national levels. A true example of the reach and influence adolescent providers have, she has contributed greatly to the advancement of adolescent health.

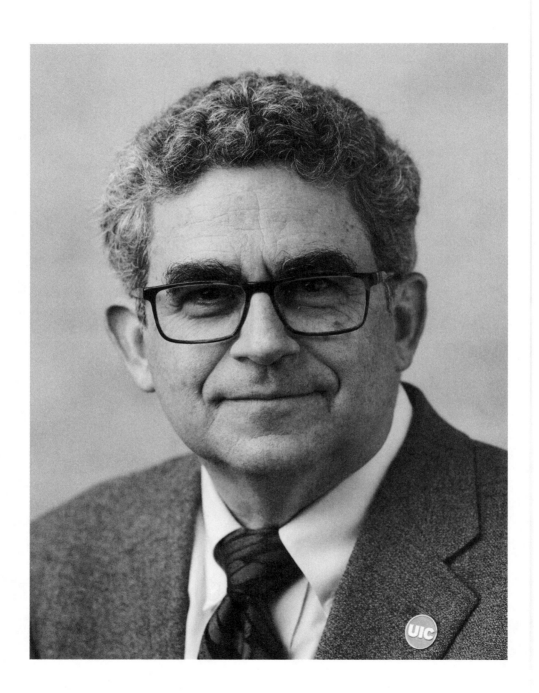

Chapter Twelve

JONATHAN D. KLEIN, MD, MPH

Jonathan Klein has devoted much of his career to addressing and improving issues of access and policy related to adolescent health. As a prominent health services researcher, he has left a strong legacy on the University of Rochester's Division of Adolescent Medicine with the work he contributed to as a faculty member from 1992 to 2009. Throughout his career, the leadership he has provided at a divisional, departmental, university, and national level through the American Academy of Pediatrics (AAP) has helped challenge and answer important questions that have contributed to advancing and improving the health of adolescents and young adults.

Klein grew up outside of New York City in a northern suburb of New Jersey and became the first person in his family to go directly to college. Though education remained important to his parents, his father enlisted in World War II the day after Pearl Harbor and then pursued his education on a part-time basis after the war ended. His mother decided later in life to continue college courses, receiving her bachelor's degree just one year before her son received his. Klein attended Brandeis University where he double majored in biology and theatre. A self-proclaimed "theatre techy," he explored his options before pursuing medicine. "Having taken a bunch of medical sociology courses, I decided that the best way to address the issues in the healthcare system, which were really interesting, would be to go to medical school," he said. He remembers Brandeis having a very socially active campus, in which students fought for many causes and where it was common for protests to occur at campus buildings. While he had a glimpse into these experiences as an undergraduate student, he became much more engaged in activism related to public health, policy, and access issues in medical school at the University of Medicine and Dentistry of New Jersey (UMDNJ). UMDNJ had some activism on the medical campus, which stood on the site of the 1960s Newark riots.

Over the course of his preclinical years, public health issues and policy really piqued his interest. He elected to pursue a Master of Public Health (MPH) degree between his third and fourth years. As he considered his best clinical fit, he says, "I think what led me to pediatrics was the sense of the ability to help young people and families transcend some of the social and economic issues." One of his mentors was Dr. Bob Johnson, an adolescent medicine physician who later became dean of UMDNJ. He introduced Dr. Klein to a multiservice center in New York City called "The Door" that offered legal aid, healthcare, education, and food services, among other needs, to the city's teenagers. "That set of experiences landed me in adolescent health and primary care and in thinking about the ways in which our system addresses access," he said.

He completed his pediatrics and chief residency at New England Medical Center in Boston, Massachusetts, before enrolling in the Robert Wood Johnson Clinical Scholars Program at the University of North Carolina at Chapel Hill, a cross-discipline fellowship in public policy and research. Throughout his fellowship, he focused on alternatives for better adolescent care and found himself interested both clinically and academically in the disparity of success in teens. After completing his fellowship, followed by two years in a junior faculty position in Chapel Hill, he and his wife, Dr. Susan Cohn (an infectious diseases physician), decided to move back to the Northeast. While they considered returning to Boston, he said he was on an elevator at a Pediatric Academic Societies (PAS) meeting with Dr. Elizabeth McAnarney and, "By the time we got off the elevator, she had convinced me to come look at Rochester."

Both he and his wife found remarkable academic job opportunities at the University of Rochester (UR) and signed on to move there for what they assumed would be four or five years, but which quickly turned into seventeen wonderful years. He was drawn to the opportunities Rochester provided him as an adolescent health services researcher, as during the early 1990s there were only a handful of these researchers across the country and several were in Rochester—thus it served as an ideal place to develop his career.

Dr. Klein remembers the strong relationship between Rochester's Divisions of Adolescent Medicine and General Pediatrics; although these were separate divisions, they were unified by both people and scholarly interests. "As a relatively small community of science, there were people who were very collaborative and also very enthusiastic about each other's work," he said. "It didn't feel at all competitive. It felt like a very supportive place to do health services research and to train people to do health services research." This relationship between the two divisions, as well as with Community and Preventive Medicine (now Public Health Sciences) and associated departments, coupled with the university's connections to the community and the ability to easily partner with the state and county, all contributed to what Dr. Klein calls "a very supportive and special environment." He also recalls strong relationships with the private practice community pediatricians in Rochester, all of whom had faculty appointments at the university. Mutual respect and collaboration fostered important interdisciplinary work and created a unique environment that allowed community pediatricians and academic researchers to work together both clinically and scholarly, a true legacy of Rochester Pediatrics. "It was a very nurturing environment for people to find those relationships and leverage them," he said. "I think there was a confluence of several factors that made both learning and teaching and doing that kind of work really easy and really rewarding in Rochester."

Dr. Klein was on the academic research track, devoting approximately 20 percent of his time to clinical work. During his time in Rochester, he had a host of roles and responsibilities, including serving as medical director for the Rochester Adolescent Maternity Program (RAMP), helping start the Teen-Tot Clinic to provide care for young mothers and their children, strengthening the fellowship program's involvement with community and school-based health centers (SBHCs), and serving as interim division chief from 2007 to 2009.

He believes one of his greatest contributions, however, was keeping an active and vigorously funded research program, for which the overriding theme was improving adolescent care delivery. His studies considered implementation of guidelines, teen pregnancy prevention, and tobacco control, as well as broader methodological studies of what kind of care adolescents were receiving and how to measure it. Throughout the years, he built a staff of research coordinators and a series of research projects with which many fellows were able to assist—many for whom he served as primary research mentor. Something of which he remains most proud in his career is the mentorship he provided to trainees, whom he said have gone on to do great things. He was also able to provide mentorship on a personal level, as many trainees looked to him and his wife, who were raising two young children at the time, as an example of how to balance family and career.

When the Division received the Leadership Education in Adolescent Health (LEAH) training grant, he played a key role with the Maternal Child Health Bureau (MCHB) related programs, as well as with the State Department of Public Health, Excellus BlueCross, and the New York State Office of Managed Care. This work in helping develop the department's governmental affairs initiatives, combined with his involvement in the American Academy of Pediatrics (AAP) and the Society for Adolescent Health and Medicine (SAHM) led to more opportunities on a national level. Dr. Michael Weitzman, who was the chief of Rochester's Division of General Pediatrics at the time, led the AAP Center for Child Health Research, which was cosponsored by the UR Department of Pediatrics. The Center formed a series of research consortia and Dr. Klein was tasked with leading the consortium focused on children and tobacco control, ultimately receiving a grant that funded the AAP's Julius B. Richmond Center.

Dr. Klein spent the last five years of his time in Rochester working with the AAP on identifying how to fund major initiatives to address significant health problems, including leading the Academy's tobacco control center. When his youngest child graduated from high school, his family moved to Chicago, where he became an Associate Executive Director of the AAP, a role he served in for seven years. He continued to work in adolescent health and tobacco control, but also had oversight for the AAP Department of Research, and for global health—an interest he particularly attributes to the influence of former UR's Department of Pediatrics chair, Dr. Robert Haggerty. Dr. Haggerty's involvement with the International Pediatric Association and other global child health groups inspired Dr. Klein's involvement with the Commonwealth Foundation's Harkness Fellowship in Healthcare Policy and Practice. Klein hosted two international fellows during his time in Rochester; an experience he says fostered his interest in comparative systems.

He is also thankful for the opportunities he had in Rochester working at the broader University and UR Medical School levels (as the Department's associate chair for Community and Government Affairs). "It definitely gave me both the skills and interest in academic governance issues and how we make medical centers and universities work for healthcare, as well as for education," he said. His career has continued in academic leadership, as he returned to an academic medical center setting at the University of Illinois at Chicago (UIC) in 2017 as a professor and executive vice head of the Department of Pediatrics, followed by becoming associate vice chancellor for Research for UIC in 2020.

Throughout his career, Dr. Klein has witnessed much growth and change in the field of adolescent medicine. However, he believes some areas remain a challenge, such as that of confidentiality, which has been one of his areas of study. He has found that twenty years ago, only about one-half of the country's teenagers had ever had private one-on-one time with their physician or other clinician. In a recent study he helped conduct, they found this number had not changed as hoped. "When we talk about all the things we should be doing in adolescent care, if we're not establishing that there is some private screening and counseling that goes on, it's really hard to do any of the things that are recommended," he said. He also notes that while interventions work, they require investment. "I think adolescents in our society still have a lot of issues in terms of what it means to grow up, and how to find meaning in your life, in your community, and in your vocation," he said, something he believes our society can improve upon.

As a specialty, Dr. Klein believes in the importance of adolescent health professionals focusing on the basic education of primary care clinicians, as well as on specialty care for young people. Since most teenagers receive care outside of a specialty setting, often by pediatricians or family medicine physicians, he said the care provided in those arenas needs to be just as good, requiring strong education during residency. He views Rochester as a place that has always had a strong cohort of adolescent medicine leaders, perhaps, he says, out of proportion to the population of the city. "We had as many adolescent medicine physicians in Rochester for most of the time that I was there than there are in the city of Chicago," he said. "And I think that brings a certain set of beliefs to training residents and training students, which is a good thing." Something else that especially stands out to him regarding Rochester's Adolescent Medicine program, is its full embracing of the biopsychosocial model. "I think Rochester Adolescent Medicine has always been a very strong voice in recognizing the biopsychosocial impact of things on young people's lives," he said. Ultimately, he says that while the "who" has changed over the years with the comings and goings of faculty, as well as the "what" of their research and scholarly interests, "their underlying commitment to the young people and to the education of clinicians in the community is the same."

Dr. Klein has spent his notable career asking important questions, advocating for adolescent health initiatives, and leading a number of prominent research and scholarly endeavors that have improved adolescent health at the local, state, national, and international levels. His leadership, mentorship, and inquiry have left an important imprint on the University of Rochester, within the Department of Pediatrics, the Division of Adolescent Medicine, the institution, and the world.

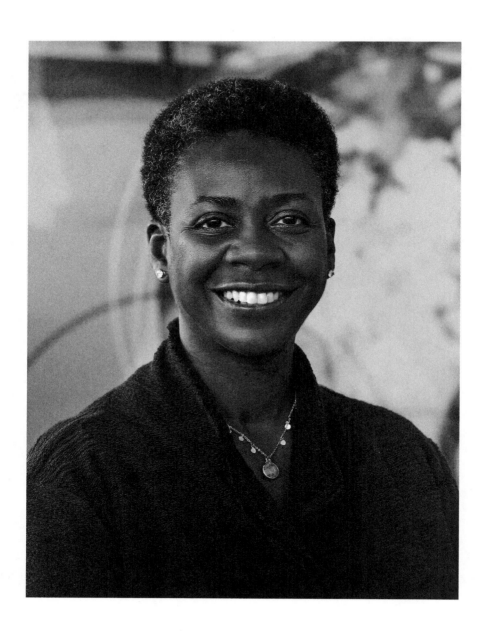

Chapter Thirteen

CHERYL M. KODJO, MD, MPH

Cheryl Kodjo has been a champion and advocate for the health of adolescents and young adults for over twenty years, spending her academic career in Rochester after graduating from the Adolescent Medicine Fellowship program in 2001. As professor of Pediatrics, an Associate Dean of Advising at the University of Rochester School of Medicine and Dentistry (URSMD), and a physician at University Health Service (UHS), Dr. Kodjo is an esteemed educator, mentor, clinician, and valued member of Rochester's Adolescent Medicine program.

Kodjo grew up in the Bronx, New York. As an educator, her father instilled the importance of education in her from a young age and encouraged her to pursue a career in medicine, a decision which she says she made by the end of high school. Her first exposure to adolescent medicine was when she was on the receiving end, which was a formative experience. She received care from a nurse practitioner who knew it was important for teenagers to be able to speak privately and confidentially with their provider, something she appreciated. Such a positive experience remained with her as she moved throughout her medical education.

She graduated from Princeton University and from Columbia University College of Physicians and Surgeons. Dr. Kodjo continued to have her initial interest in caring for adolescents, while simultaneously realizing she knew little about teenagers. She thought seriously about her ultimate career goals. In medical school, she pursued elective opportunities to gain more experience in caring for adolescents. Columbia had an affiliation with Harlem Hospital, which had a very active primary care practice for adolescents. She completed an elective experience there and found she was drawn to the counseling aspect of the field. "I will always say I'm not a therapist," she said, "but there is something to be said for listening and letting patients feel heard, providing support and options. I liked that aspect of care."

Knowing early on that she wanted to go into pediatrics, she completed her residency at Albert Einstein College of Medicine in the Bronx, during which time she continued to pursue electives in adolescent medicine. During that time, adolescent medicine was not a required rotation (something that has since changed for today's pediatric residents). "A distinct learning experience in adolescent medicine facilitates understanding the nuances of adolescent growth and development," Dr. Kodjo said. "I'm happy to see the progress in medical education over time and that the trainees understand the uniqueness of adolescent development. Whether one is planning on becoming a general pediatrician or a subspecialist, a working understanding of adolescent development is critically important in providing care to this population."

When it came time to apply for fellowship, Dr. Kodjo applied to the University of Rochester from a recommendation she received from a fellow at Albert Einstein. This fellow went to medical school at the University of Rochester and was taught by Drs. Elizabeth McAnarney and Richard Kreipe, the then-department chair of Pediatrics and division chief of Adolescent Medicine, respectively. This fellow respected them and regarded the fellowship program highly. Dr. Kodjo received that same impression of the program upon her interview and believed it would support and foster her interests, which at the time were teen pregnancy and primary care for adolescents.

Dr. Kodjo began her adolescent medicine fellowship in 1998 in Rochester as part of the second cohort of the program's Leadership Education in Adolescent Health (LEAH) training program. Even today, she continues to value her experience with the LEAH program. "That exposure of working with colleagues from different disciplines and gaining a better understanding of what they do and what skills they have in providing comprehensive care were very formative," she recalls. The work was rewarding. "Working with teenagers and their families can be challenging. Thus, it is critical that a team of professionals oversee their care. It was always invigorating to hear the insights of providers of different backgrounds and to think creatively on how to approach different challenges," she said. Dr. Kodjo's involvement with the LEAH program continued after she graduated, as she served as the medicine discipline coordinator and training director for a number of years. She remains close with many of her LEAH colleagues across disciplines to this day.

Dr. Kodjo chose to remain in Rochester following her fellowship and she assumed different leadership roles in the division, department, and institution. Working closely with nurse practitioner Jane Tuttle, PhD, FNP, she assumed the role of medical director of the hospital's Teen-Tot clinic. Although portions of the program were developed in the mid-1970s, this "new" clinic was started by Dr. Tuttle and a former adolescent medicine fellow, Dr. Laurie Mitan, in the early-to-mid 1990s, a time of high teenage pregnancy rates in Rochester. They partnered with the Rochester Adolescent Maternity Program (RAMP), from whom many of these patients were receiving their prenatal care. RAMP staff could direct these young patients to the Teen-Tot clinic, whose providers would then provide medical care for mother and baby in one setting. In addition, the clinic provided primary care to adolescents who were nonmothers, including adolescents who needed school/sports physicals, contraception, sexually transmitted infection (STI) screening, and risk assessments. The site served as the only on-site general pediatrics practice to care for young people ages birth to twenty-one within the Division of Adolescent Medicine.

Throughout her career, Dr. Kodjo has witnessed a national dialogue occur in the field as to whether the nature of adolescent medicine is and should be a subspecialty or primary care. While Rochester has renowned subspecialty services, with premier eating disorder, gender health, and reproductive health programs, this primary care presence was important to her. Dr. Kodjo believes a strong community presence is very important in order to meet adolescents where they are and to allow for early intervention in a young person's development. The clinic remained a strong educational site for medical students, residents, and fellows to rotate through 2017 when Dr. Tuttle retired and Dr. Kodjo began her practice at UHS.

Another early interest of Dr. Kodjo's was that of mental health. She remembers Dr. McAnarney reflecting that mental health was the new crisis in pediatrics, something that nearly twenty years later she believes has not changed. "It's no longer new, it has been a crisis in pediatrics and every other primary care specialty," she said. She became interested in this topic during her fellowship in the late 1990s, a time when mass school shootings were becoming more prevalent. Her research during fellowship and in her early years as a faculty member was to understand the risk factors that helped create an individual who would engage in such behavior. Using national databases, she studied barriers to mental health and predictors of depression, ultimately leading her to receive a small departmental grant that allowed her to go into the Rochester City School District to speak directly with students about mental health care.

The importance of mental health has remained an interest and played an important role throughout her career, perhaps even more so in recent times as she worked with undergraduate and graduate students on the University of Rochester's River Campus during the unprecedented time of the COVID-19 pandemic. She brings a unique perspective as an adolescent medicine physician at UHS, as she notes that mental health continues to be the number one issue that is problematic on college campuses. "Mental health is huge within this population. Being really creative about how to help adolescents and young adults to negotiate personal, familial, and societal issues and emerge as healthy adults is our challenge," she said. Dr. Kodjo has found ample opportunities to provide general counseling and support during the challenging and unprecedented times of the pandemic, which required the need for virtual learning and social distancing (counter to optimum adolescent and young adult development), and the anxiety-provoking national climate resulting from the pandemic and racial unrest.

Her counseling and support extend to URSMD, where she has served as an advisory dean to medical students since 2008. Her first introduction to the medical school was in 2004 when a senior colleague encouraged her to work as part of the School of Medicine's Diversity Theme Committee, of which she served as director for a number of years. With the encouragement of this colleague and support from Dr. Kreipe, she received a National Heart, Lung, and Blood Institute (NHLBI) grant, the focus of which was cultural competency education. This was a time when the medical school was being held more accountable by its licensing body for cultural competency training, so she was able to become immersed in the medical school to not only teach herself, but to look at different curricular pieces, which she believes to have been a very serendipitous time in her career.

Through this work with the medical school, she became increasingly interested in pursuing an advisory dean position. She discussed this interest with the senior associate dean and, when a position became available, she was offered the opportunity. When explaining this multifaceted role, she said, "The easy pass at the question is that we oversee the professional development and career advising of our assigned students." In reality, she spends her time at the medical school addressing a broad array of student concerns, ranging from course remediation and a change in heart around specialty choices to reviewing residency application materials and summer plans to student health and well-being. It is a busy, all-encompassing job, but one that she enjoys. She says she has a great team at the medical school, which replicates her experience in Adolescent Medicine. "As long as the team is good, even though there are difficult circumstances, you can always get recentered and reenergized."

Dr. Kodjo is most proud of her mentoring relationships, particularly with former fellows and other trainees who have careers working or interfacing with adolescents in the division and around the country. In 2005, along with Dr. Lee Pachter, she served as a cofounder of a mentoring program through the Academic Pediatric Association (APA) called the New Century Scholars Program, a national role she held for ten years. This program sought to increase workforce diversity by encouraging trainees of color and/or with an interest in health equity to consider academic fellowships. A multitiered program mentoring all levels, from fellow to faculty, it is ongoing today. She is proud to have taken part in such an initiative that inspired a number of people to pursue careers in academic pediatrics, including adolescent medicine—many of whom have gone on to be influential in their fields.

Reflecting on the future of adolescent medicine, Dr. Kodjo believes the field often follows major recent social movements, which she has seen most recently in the LGBTQ+ and gender identity movements, which have greatly influenced practices. With the racial inequities and recent unrest surfacing in the summer of 2020, she thinks racial equity will be the next frontier. "It's what young people are concerned about and what is on their minds," she said.

Dr. Kodjo has seen the field, locally and nationally, undergo changes over the years and looks forward to continuing to witness how it will grow and evolve. She is a strong leader and role model who is providing insights, talents, and passion to the field and has contributed greatly to the University of Rochester as an institution, its Adolescent Medicine program, the students and trainees she has mentored and supported, and the countless patients and families for whom she has cared throughout her career.

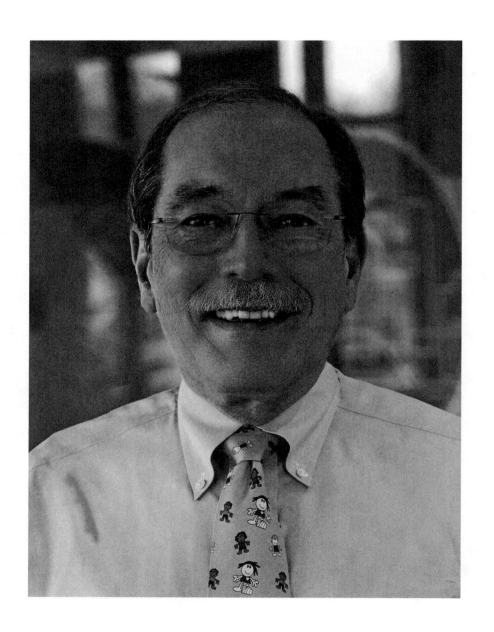

Chapter Fourteen

Richard E. Kreipe, MD

One cannot discuss adolescent medicine and eating disorder treatment and care without recognizing Richard E. Kreipe. As a national leader, renowned clinician, and beloved colleague, Dr. Kreipe, now professor emeritus, has left a strong legacy in the field, making significant contributions to adolescent health throughout the past forty-plus years.

Born in Oklahoma, his father's career as a chemical engineer moved the family around until they settled in Philadelphia, Pennsylvania, when Rich was five years old. While he was the first person in his family to pursue medicine, he said he learned the value of hard work from his father. His paternal grandfather, a farmer in Kansas, died at the age of twenty-five in the 1918 influenza epidemic, which left Rich's father as the "man-of-the-house" at the age of three. By simultaneously working on the farm and earning his chemical engineering degree from the University of Kansas, his father served as a great inspiration.

Kreipe attended LaSalle College in Philadelphia for his undergraduate education, where he majored in biology. He was always interested in science and thought he would become an ecologist during the time when pollution was just starting to be studied—in fact, he celebrated the very first Earth Day (April 22, 1970) while sitting in a college ecology class. During his junior year, he conducted research that identified an organism in a small stream that blooms when there is toxic effluent from paper manufacturing. He laughs, saying he thought he was going to spend his career "throwing polluters in jail to save Mother Earth."

However, when he told a biology professor this plan, that professor told him he would need to get a PhD "if he didn't want to just be rowing some scientist around in a boat," which could take a minimum of five years, after which some people would not finish at all. Having second thoughts, Kreipe asked the professor what he thought he should do. "I think you should be a physician," he said. When Kreipe asked him why, he said, "Because I think you'd be a good one." He applied to only two medical schools in Philadelphia—his thought being that if he did not get in, he would take the entrance examination for graduate school. He was admitted to both and decided to attend Temple University.

During medical school he was drawn to pediatrics and, when it came time to apply for residency, he chose to stay in Philadelphia and attend St. Christopher's Hospital for Children, the third oldest children's hospital in the country. However, he also applied to the University of Rochester, which was his first introduction to Dr. Elizabeth McAnarney, when she interviewed him. While he did not go to Rochester for residency, he said he always kept Dr. McAnarney in the back of his mind, especially as he found himself gravitating toward adolescent medicine and he knew Rochester had an extremely strong program. "I remember when I interviewed for my internship with Lissa McAnarney, I said, 'That's the person I want to train with.' She's got the kind of energy that I wanted to be surrounded by."

With his sights set on fellowship in Rochester, he was offered a chief resident position at St. Christopher's. It was Dr. McAnarney who gave him the sage advice that he would only have one chance to do a chief residency and assured him there would be a spot in the fellowship program waiting for him the following year. He accepted the chief resident position and is grateful for that experience.

Two weeks before he was leaving for Rochester, he was conducting chief rounds with a group of residents and medical students when they stopped at a single room occupied by a young, very thin female patient. When Dr. Kreipe put his hand on the doorknob, he was warned not to go inside. When he asked why not, he was told that the patient had anorexia nervosa. He immediately pulled his hand away and said, "Is she contagious?" "Four years of medical school, three years of residency, and one year minus two weeks of chief residency and I had never heard those words," he said. He was told that the patient had a psychiatric illness and they shouldn't go into the patient's room—a statement he said was further explained by an inaccurate and massive generalization that patients with anorexia nervosa are manipulative, will lie, and tend to have complicated family relationships. While he moved on from this first experience with the condition, little did he know he would encounter an adolescent who had the same illness again in just two short weeks as an adolescent medicine fellow in Rochester, when he met his first patient there who had anorexia nervosa.

He remembers this encounter clearly and approached it with humility, admitting to the patient that he had never treated anyone who had anorexia nervosa and that the first time he heard the term was just two weeks previously, so he would need her to help him understand more about her illness. He said he fully acknowledged to her that she could both feel fat (just like she could feel happy or sad) and also be medically sick from being too thin, and between those two truths was where the disorder lived. "I learned that accepting the patient where she was is an important principle of adolescent medicine," he said. "It's important in all medical care, but especially adolescents—not judging them." Further, he believes that the then-dominant "psychiatric" model of anorexia nervosa tended to blame parents and patients, which he found to be neither accurate nor helpful.

On the basis of his clinical observation, he began to examine the condition from a developmental perspective. "That was a unique way of evaluating the young patient's circumstances, as the traditional model at the time was that the majority of the condition was psychological with little consideration of the broader biopsychosocial perspective and related conditions," he said. "The approach of 'What's wrong with you' regarding psychological symptoms and not considering the adolescent's developmental age and vulnerabilities and often medical fragility *as a result* of the underlying psychological symptoms, in my mind, was short-sighted." He believes adolescents already tend to be self-critical; there is no need for someone in a helping profession to add to the criticism. Having devoted most of his career to positive youth development as a public health framework for common adolescent health concerns at the local, state, national, and global level, he said, "I firmly believe in a strength-based approach." It was this perspective that would lead Dr. Kreipe to make remarkable progress in changing the conceptualization of the illness to be a developmental challenge, rather than a purely psychological one.

Upon completion of his fellowship, the then chair of the Department of Pediatrics, Dr. David H. Smith, asked Dr. Kreipe to stay on for a one-year position to cover Dr. McAnarney's duties while she completed a sabbatical at Cornell University. He became the acting medical director of the Rochester Adolescent Maternity Program (RAMP). He also was tasked with starting an Adolescent Medicine ambulatory program at Rochester General Hospital (RGH). When he originally came to Rochester in 1979, he thought that he would remain for only his two-year fellowship before immediately returning to Philadelphia "because who could live in Rochester for more than two years?" he said with a laugh. However, he felt so supported in his young academic career and accepted the position to stay. What started as a one-year position turned into a 41-year fruitful career!

In addition to the important contributions that he has made and continues to make in the evolution of the conceptualization of anorexia nervosa as a developmental condition, Dr. Kreipe's career is one filled with accomplishments and leadership that has led to transformative advances and improvements in adolescent health care nationally and internationally. In 1985, he developed the University of Rochester's Child and Adolescent Eating Disorder Program, which remains a strong and renowned program today. In 1990, he coedited the *Textbook of Adolescent Medicine* with Drs. McAnarney, Donald Orr (a former University of Rochester fellow), and George Comerci (American Academy of Pediatrics [AAP] former president), followed by the *Textbook of Adolescent Health Care* published by the AAP in 2011. In 1993, following Dr. McAnarney's 22-year tenure as chief of the Division of Adolescent Medicine, he assumed the role of division chief, a role in which he served for fourteen years. He was also the founding medical director of the Western New York Comprehensive Care Center for Eating Disorders.

Dr. Kreipe later served as President of the Society for Adolescent Medicine (SAM) from 2008 to 2009. Dr. Kreipe was the fifth president to come from the University of Rochester, a strong legacy of which he was honored to become a part. His last official act as president was recognizing finally the interprofessional nature of the organization by voting to change its name to the Society for Adolescent *Health* and Medicine (SAHM).

Dr. Kreipe believes that one of his greatest contributions occurred in 1997, when he successfully competed for one of only six federally funded Leadership Education in Adolescent Health (LEAH) interdisciplinary training grants. The University of Rochester had degree-granting programs for only three of the five core disciplines—medicine, nursing, and psychology—but Dr. Kreipe had the vision to partner with other area universities to create an upstate coalition. He collaborated with Cornell University, which had a world-famous nutrition program, and Syracuse University, which had a leadership program in social work funded by the Maternal and Child Health Bureau (MCHB). This collaboration led to fifteen years of continuous federal funding totaling more than $6,000,000. Dr. Kreipe served as the director of the LEAH program throughout those fifteen years, training dozens of future leaders, several of whom are featured in this book.

Another pivotal moment occurred for Dr. Kreipe in 2008 when he was asked to join the eating disorder workgroup for the American Psychiatric Association's fifth edition of the *Diagnostic and Statistical Manual* (*DSM-5*), as the only pediatrician or adolescent medicine specialist. He can remember arriving at the first meeting in Arlington, Virginia, and being surrounded by the major leaders in the eating disorder world. He humbly recounts looking at the icons in the room and feeling as if he didn't belong in this esteemed group. He could see the airport just outside the window, and realizing it was no more than a mile away, pondered if he should get on a plane back to Rochester. "I was close to doing that, but my conscience says, 'No, Kreipe, you need to be here to speak on behalf of adolescent patients and their parents,'" he said.

The discussion began with the criteria for anorexia nervosa, for which the first criterion began "Refusal to maintain a minimal normal weight." Dr. Kreipe asked the group why the first word was "refusal," a pejorative term that immediately identifies the patient as being oppositional, not cooperative. "How do you establish a therapeutic relationship with a patient when you automatically identify them as doing the opposite of what you want them to do?" he said. This conversation sparked a change, and in the *DSM-5*'s criteria the words were changed to "restriction of caloric intake." He also pushed back on the term *Ideal Body Weight* and advocated for the removal of all weight thresholds in the diagnosis. "It was like I sucked all the air out of the room," he said. He had seen firsthand the lengths patients would go to in order to "make weight" and avoid admittance into the hospital—for example, one patient who drank an excessive amount of water the morning of her appointment. While the number on the scale reflected "health," her physical examination did not. With decreased blood sodium levels from extreme, rapid water loading, she had put herself at risk for a seizure. Dr. Kreipe's advocacy for patients who had anorexia nervosa resulted in the elimination of any mention of weight thresholds in the diagnosis of anorexia nervosa in the *DSM-5*, which has shifted the focus to parameters of health rather than numbers on a scale. This is the contribution to his field of which he is most proud.

Throughout Dr. Kreipe's career, he has integrated the biopsychosocial model into the care of his patients, a model developed in Rochester and which he believes is at the heart of the Rochester Adolescent Medicine program. It is a program he finds to be a combination of expert clinical care with strong training in the community, success in clinically oriented research that considers ways of improving care, but with a powerful academic foundation, and one which can be described by "excellence," "curiosity more than certainty," and "hope."

Dr. Kreipe has much hope for the future of adolescent medicine and attributes the potential for the field to the young professionals entering it who have bright, committed, energetic minds. As he reflects, he draws a parallel to his early interest in ecology—"The most appropriate view of human growth and development is an ecological one," he said, citing Cornell Professor Urie Bronfenbrenner, who coined the term *human ecology* to highlight the dynamic interaction between humans and their environment. "The state of adolescent health is much more determined by those larger influences … however, I have always emphasized that an individual professional in the field can have a very important influence on changing the life course of individual adolescents with whom they work." Dr. Kreipe is a true testament to that, as he has touched the lives of many. He has numerous patients who have kept in touch with him over the years, even inviting him to their weddings.

Through Dr. Kreipe's leadership, which has extended internationally, the education he has provided to generations of adolescent health providers, his perspectives on patient care and positive youth development that have brought about important change, and the bonds he has created with his patients and colleagues, he has left not only a long-lasting legacy for the Rochester program, but he has truly improved the field of adolescent medicine and the health of adolescents throughout the world.

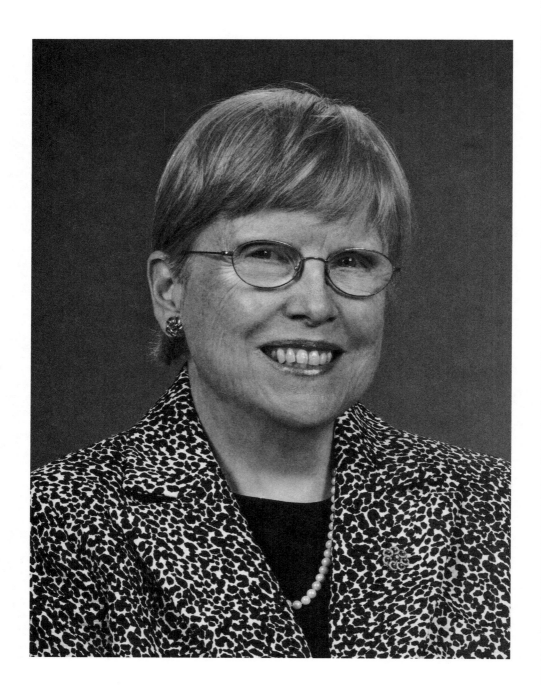

Chapter Fifteen

Elizabeth R. McAnarney, MD

The University of Rochester's Department of Pediatrics Adolescent Medicine Program is one of the oldest in the country, dating back to the early 1960s. Elizabeth (Lissa) McAnarney served as one of its earliest leaders, transforming it from a once-a-week clinic to a clinically and scientifically robust program and official division, well respected across the institution and nation. As one of the early developers of the field itself, Dr. McAnarney has been a prominent leader for over fifty years, devoting her remarkable career to improving child and adolescent health. She led the Adolescent Medicine program for twenty-two years, followed by serving as chair of Pediatrics for thirteen years. A national and international leader, she is a past president of the Society for Adolescent Health and Medicine (SAHM), the American Pediatric Society (APS) and the first woman to serve as president of the Association of Medical School Pediatric Chairs. She received the prestigious John Howland Lifetime Achievement Award from the APS. A true pioneer in the field of adolescent medicine, she conducted seminal research on adolescent pregnancy, developed one of the first national adolescent medicine curriculums, and has been involved with each major milestone from the field's early development to receiving board recognition, to becoming a valued subspecialty truly integrated into pediatric healthcare.

Dr. McAnarney has a longstanding interest in working with children and studied as an undergraduate in a prominent child development program. Her interest in adolescents developed during her senior undergraduate seminar when she helped annotate and update the bibliography of a well-known child development book. She was tasked with editing the section on adolescence.

As she applied to medical school, she was encouraged to study with Dr. Julius B. Richmond. Dr. Richmond was the chair of Pediatrics at Syracuse at the time and would later go on to become the Surgeon General under former President Jimmy Carter.

She remained in Syracuse for her residency training in pediatrics. It was the mid-1960s, which she remembers as a time when many pediatric disease prognoses were dire. Conditions for which the prognosis for the children was not good were congenital heart disease, cystic fibrosis (CF), and acute lymphoblastic leukemia (ALL), among others; life expectancies for children who had these conditions were extremely low. Some who had congenital diseases died right after birth and others died in early childhood; for example, it was remarkable if children who had CF lived until age ten, and nearly 80% of children with ALL did not survive. These numbers have improved drastically over the years, with many surviving CF well into adulthood and 90% of children now surviving ALL. However, after two years of experiencing such loss in residency, Dr. McAnarney thoughtfully considered her next step. "I would love to see well children, but the loss of a child was so frequent that I thought that would be very difficult," she said. She also continued to develop her interest in adolescent medicine during residency, as she would often trade inpatient rotations with her coresidents who did not want to care for adolescents, trading her other rotations for more time spent in adolescent clinic.

Dr. Richmond encouraged her to apply to the University of Rochester (UR) to study with Dr. Robert Haggerty, the third chair of the UR Department of Pediatrics who cofounded behavioral pediatrics at Rochester. As fate would have it, Dr. Haggerty was presenting at Grand Rounds at Syracuse in the last year of Dr. McAnarney's residency. Dr. Haggerty really impressed her with his insightful and clairvoyant message that children's behavioral problems would emerge and grow over time. She recalls Dr. Haggerty presenting the clear picture of the future of pediatrics—a world in which vaccines and antibiotics would reduce the incidence of infectious disease and where there would be better treatment for children who had leukemia. He prophesied that the conditions that would remain would be congenital conditions, and an increasing presence of social and behavioral problems. "The concepts Dr. Haggerty developed in the mid-1960s are now coming to fruition," she said.

In 1968, Dr. McAnarney arrived in Rochester to pursue a behavioral pediatrics fellowship with Dr. Haggerty and Dr. Stanford B. Friedman, who trained at Massachusetts General Hospital and worked with a leading psychiatrist at the National Institutes of Mental Health (NIMH). Both Drs. Friedman and Haggerty believed that psychosocial issues affected children's development and biological status. Both had trained with Dr. George Engel, who developed the biopsychosocial model of medicine in Rochester. McAnarney was the third fellow in the behavioral pediatrics program and it was during that time that she continued to cultivate her interest in adolescent medicine.

When Dr. McAnarney assumed the directorship of the Adolescent Medicine program over fifty years ago, it was a weekly clinic that met on Saturday mornings (the only time that there was ambulatory space in the hospital). Dr. Friedman strongly believed in interdisciplinary care, and the clinic was inclusive of colleagues from nursing, social work, and medicine. "We had a terrific sense of spirit and unity, and the patient and family were the focuses," Dr. McAnarney said. She describes Dr. Friedman as a "super trainer of the fellows" and "available, knowledgeable, and a great advocate for adolescents." Another mentor for her was Dr. Christopher Hodgman, a beloved adult psychiatrist who served in the clinic regularly. "He was a doctor's doctor," Dr. McAnarney said. She remembers Dr. Hodgman saying that if there are psychiatric illnesses that present the same way patient after patient, there is probably a biologic basis for the condition. He believed this to be true for eating disorders, but many disagreed with him, believing almost entirely in Freudian theory at that time. As science has revealed the important relationships between the neurologic system and behavior, Dr. Hodgman's beliefs have become widely accepted.

It was during Dr. McAnarney's third year of fellowship that Dr. Haggerty asked her to become the director of the Adolescent Medicine program. She remembers responding to Dr. Haggerty with appreciation and saying, "We don't have a program—we have a one-day clinic, there is no science, and there is no field. I'm taking a big academic risk." To which he said, "No risk, no gain, Lissa." Thus, in 1972, she embarked on a journey in adolescent medicine that would be marked with profound growth, challenges along the way, but many rewards. She remembers other physicians and administrators being very skeptical about creating a special emphasis on the health of adolescents, as adolescent medicine did not exist in the eyes of the institution, pediatricians, or subspecialists at that time. "There was no field of adolescent medicine. It was poorly reimbursed and we had much resistance," she said, remembering thinking, "What have I gotten myself into? I'm out in this ocean with barely a boat!" However, she approached the challenge head on, utilizing her guiding principles of leadership.

Her first principle was to become an academically and community-wide responsible field. She knew that if she were to lead a group of colleagues in an academic setting, she had to fully understand and communicate the rules/principles for academic promotion, and that everyone had to play by the same rules of the game as colleagues in every other subspecialty. "If you want to integrate into the whole, you have to play by the rules," she said. She also had to build a program/division based on excellence in everything undertaken.

Second, utilize the clinical program as a laboratory. She felt strongly that every clinical program in an academic setting should have a strong research component. Her clinical laboratory became that of the Rochester Adolescent Maternity Program (RAMP), where she conducted seminal research on adolescent pregnancy, which resulted in nationally and internationally known findings that mother's age alone did not predestine her to have a small baby. Rather, if given the proper medical and psychosocial care, the outcomes of adolescent mothers and their babies are positive.

Third, attend academic conferences at the national level—attend meetings, present high-quality research often, and ensure trainees are actively involved in meeting national colleagues and learning to present their research findings and develop their identities nationally. Dr. McAnarney joined the Society for Adolescent Health and Medicine (SAHM), then the nascent Society for Adolescent Medicine (SAM), when there were only 35–40 members. The attendees became the group of people ultimately responsible for creating the field of adolescent medicine. "We always took our trainees with us to the meetings so they could see the opportunity for them to create the field with us," she said. Through Dr. McAnarney's early involvement with SAHM, she became responsible with a team of others for creating the first national curriculum in adolescent medicine. In the early 1990s, the "pioneers" including

Dr. McAnarney were involved in the development of receiving official subspecialty board recognition of adolescent medicine from the American Board of Pediatrics (ABP). "We realized that we should extend national participation in organizations outside of SAHM to leverage their help to connect to an even wider audience," she said. She and several others from SAHM became active with the American Academy of Pediatrics (AAP). Dr. McAnarney served as one of the earlier chairs of the newly created Section of Adolescent Health and the Committee on Pediatric Research early on in her tenure. She credits the AAP's endorsement of adolescent medicine among the national AAP members and leadership as a major contributor to the growth of the field of adolescent medicine.

Another principle was to grasp the imaginations of the students and residents. She understood the importance of interesting young trainees in the field. At the beginning of her tenure when the program could rent space from the hospital only on Saturdays and evenings, Dr. McAnarney personally approached each resident and asked if he or she would like to help cover these clinics. She knew that adolescents were underrepresented in the medical system and that the providers were uncomfortable caring for them. "The residents learned that adolescents had similar needs medically and behaviorally as children, and that they were like every other patient for whom we cared, even though sometimes they were challenging," she said. "So, we really tried to get the students and the residents to be the advocates for adolescents and they did a wonderful job. We groomed them to be future leaders in the field. I'm so proud of our trainees, many of whom are featured in this book. They have accomplished so much on behalf of adolescents' and their families' well-being."

Another principle for a struggling new field was to be available 24/7 for clinical questions and care. During the first three years of her directorship, Dr. McAnarney was the sole faculty member in Adolescent Medicine. Dr. O.J. Sahler returned to Rochester for her fellowship training three years later, and Dr. Donald Orr also joined at the same time as a fellow, having studied adolescent medicine for a year at the University of Colorado.

The evolution of the program during Dr. McAnarney's twenty-two years of leadership was remarkable. What began as a once-a-week Saturday morning clinic and inpatient consultation program expanded to include RAMP, and later extended into the community through operating the youth center, Threshold. It was in the mid-1970s that plans for the new hospital were being developed and Dr. McAnarney persistently approached Dr. Haggerty to request an adolescent inpatient unit—a unit specifically designed for teenagers consisting of all of the interdisciplinary services needed. There was skepticism at the hospital level, but as Dr. Haggerty was leaving to go on sabbatical, he gave Dr. McAnarney permission to move forward. She personally went to the construction site and assigned space to Adolescent Medicine, and when the new hospital opened, her dream of having a dedicated adolescent inpatient unit was realized. "That gave us a site in which to be noticed and where the optimal care of adolescents was being provided," she said. The majority of adolescents who were between the ages of twelve to twenty-one who had primarily medical diagnoses were hospitalized there. It was on this unit that Rochester's nationally renowned Eating Disorder Program was created, primarily led by Dr. Richard Kreipe. Dr. McAnarney notes that previously patients who had eating disorders were typically housed in the inpatient unit in psychiatry. Dr. McAnarney encouraged Dr. Kreipe to use the adolescent unit as his clinical laboratory. He went on to receive national and international recognition for his work focused on adolescents who have eating disorders.

Dr. McAnarney is proud of fact that the majority of the programs developed in the 1960s and 1970s within the Rochester program have continued to this day. She is thankful for the mentors, colleagues, and trainees that were a major part of the journey. This includes the early support of Drs. Friedman, Haggerty, and Hodgman; her administrator of forty-seven years, Carole Berger, to whom this book is dedicated; each of the fellows who shared their talents; and the program's influential nurse leader, Marilyn Aten, PhD, RN, who was instrumental in creating RAMP and the inpatient unit. "We also had very special people within the institution who supported us when few others did. They were strong professionals whose sole interest professionally was on the best interests of the adolescents and their families. Our advocacy took us deep into the community—adolescents' homes, the Monroe County Department of Health, the courts, houses of worship, schools, impoverished neighborhoods, and wherever there were adolescents in need of care." she said. Colleagues from outside the programs also included Dr. Gary Myers, a pediatric neurologist who routinely brought his adolescent patients who had seizures to the adolescent clinic for care as well as training of the young; Dr. Gilbert Forbes, who shared his insights from his prominent research on growth and expertise in adolescence; and Dr. Henry Thiede, the chair of Obstetrics and Gynecology, who was supportive of Dr. McAnarney and the program's efforts in RAMP. Dr. Thiede also introduced the concept of nurse midwives to the hospital, the most prominent and long-serving were Ms. Beth Cooper and Ms. Helene Thompson-Scott (see Chapter 25). The nurse midwife model of care was ideal for the young pregnant adolescent as the adolescents mostly did not require subspecialty medical care, but needed mostly routine prenatal care. The patients really liked working with the midwives who provided not only excellent prenatal care, but also ideal female role models.

Final reflections that Dr. McAnarney shared as she moves into six decades in the field: "Build relationships with other people and programs. Assure dignity and integrity in every aspect of the program. Lead with kindness and thoughtful loyalty. Enjoy the creativity of adolescents and those attracted to provide care for them. Take strategic chances. Look for those people who are friends and who will be honest with you and reflect with you as to what is working and not working (that includes the adolescent patients and their families—our consumer evaluations were helpful in modifying our programs). And the last one is, create, create, and create. Love being a doctor, and have gratitude."

Dr. McAnarney has had the unique opportunity to watch the development of the field of adolescent medicine from its earliest days, and to not only witness it, but to be a key contributor and force in that growth. Receiving the designation as a Distinguished University Professor, she has a strong legacy at the University of Rochester—within the institution, Department of Pediatrics, Division of Adolescent Medicine, and greater community. An influential leader, beloved mentor, and inspiring trailblazer, her legacy is also deeply felt within the field of adolescent medicine—a field that exists in large part due to the vision, dedication, and tireless work of its early creators.

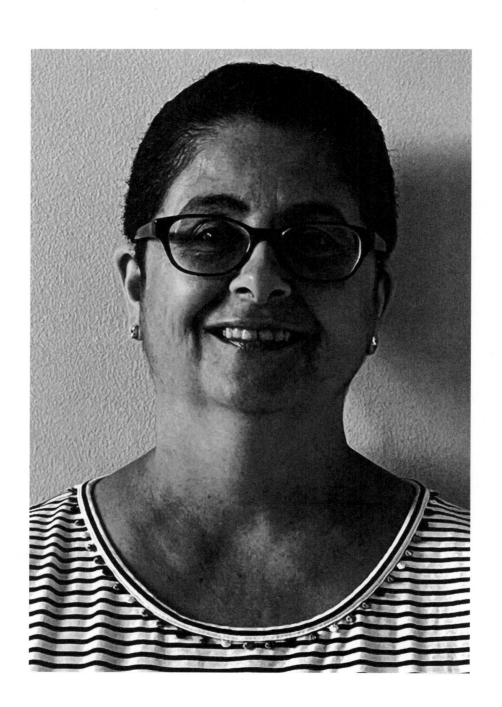

Chapter Sixteen

LAURIE A. MITAN, MD, FAAP

Laurie Mitan has dedicated much of her inspiring career to caring for adolescents who have eating disorders. A leader in the field, she has built a robust and esteemed eating disorder program from the ground up at her current institution, Cincinnati Children's Hospital, where she serves as associate professor of Pediatrics and medical director of the Eating Disorder Program. A 1996 graduate of the University of Rochester Adolescent Medicine Fellowship program, she is grateful for her experience and the start it gave her, providing much of the foundation and introduction to her work with adolescents who have eating disorders.

Mitan grew up in Suffolk County on Long Island, New York. She remembers her interest in medicine beginning as early as in the eighth grade, when she interviewed her pediatrician for a class assignment. She admired the way he helped people, and from then on, she aspired to become a physician. "I just set my sights on that and never blinked," she said. She attended Creighton University in Omaha, Nebraska, for her undergraduate and medical education before heading back East for her pediatric residency, which she completed at State University of New York (SUNY) Upstate in Syracuse, New York. Added advantages for Dr. Mitan in going to SUNY Upstate were that her sister was living in Syracuse and her husband was able to complete his master's in social work (MSW) at Syracuse University.

When it was time for Dr. Mitan to apply for an adolescent medicine fellowship, she interviewed at the University of Rochester and immediately fell in love with the program and its leaders. Her initial interest was in adolescent pregnancy, thus the Rochester Adolescent Maternity Program (RAMP) and Dr.

Elizabeth McAnarney's leadership were of great interest to her. During the time of her interview, Dr. McAnarney was the division chief of Adolescent Medicine; however, soon after she accepted the position of chair of the Department of Pediatrics. "Dr. McAnarney's ethics, moral code, and mentorship were so strong that she personally called me to tell me about the leadership change to make sure I weighed that in my decision," Dr. Mitan said. Dr. McAnarney knew of Dr. Mitan's interest in adolescent pregnancy and explained that while she would still have a strong presence in that area, it would look different from what they had originally discussed. "I really think her professionalism couldn't be beaten and was one of the strongest reasons I chose the Rochester program over some of the others that also had a teen pregnancy focus. I chose people over the particular subject matter," she said with a smile.

Dr. Mitan has the fondest memories of her fellowship and oftentimes finds herself utilizing those memories and experiences to help guide the fellowship program at her current institution. She said any credentialed fellowship program is going to provide great teaching, but Rochester had this added element of the "personal touch." She remembers sharing an office with her two cofellows, which furthered the camaraderie that the program fostered. "They really encouraged fellowship bonding, teamwork, and support. The senior fellows helped the junior fellows and there wasn't any flavor at all of competition," she said. She remains grateful for the personal interest Dr. McAnarney took in the adolescent medicine fellows while she was chair of a busy Department of Pediatrics, remembering Dr. McAnarney stopping by their office on Friday afternoons, inviting them to tea, and even giving Dr. Mitan the opportunity to review a journal article with her. This camaraderie extended throughout the whole division, Dr. Mitan remembers, describing Rochester as a "family-oriented training program." She vividly remembers sitting in Dr. Richard Kreipe's office with all the adolescent medicine faculty and fellows, presenting patients and talking through issues with difficult patients—a very helpful and valuable aspect of her training. "It was like a family meeting," she said. "When I think of Rochester, I think of the wonderful people who were great mentors, colleagues, and friends."

During fellowship, Dr. Mitan utilized her sociology background and became interested in the psychosocial aspects of adolescent pregnancy, including the relationships between teenage parents. It was this interest that led her into the community, specifically to the Anthony Jordan Health Center, where she gained much insight into the struggles of adolescent mothers and fathers. This experience inspired her to envision a clinical endeavor that would help relieve some of their stress by offering a one-stop clinic that would care for both mother and baby—thus, the Teen-Tot clinic was born. She worked with Dr. Jane Tuttle who kept the clinic running after Dr. Mitan's graduation, ultimately developing it over the next twenty plus years as a key clinical practice of the division, department, and children's hospital.

Upon Dr. Mitan's graduation from fellowship, she accepted a position at Vanderbilt University. Due to the small size of its clinical program, she was unable to narrow her focus to solely teenage parents, and had a broad range of clinical duties. She loved working at the Vanderbilt undergraduate campus health center primarily focusing on eating disorders and gynecological care. As her interest continued to grow, she devoted more of her time there, until she received a call one day from Dr. Gail Slap, the newly appointed division chief of Adolescent Medicine at the University of Cincinnati College of Medicine/Cincinnati Children's Hospital. One of Dr. Slap's primary goals was to expand eating disorder care, which was a request from the community and not a focus of the division at the time. Dr. Slap received Dr. Mitan's name and strong recommendation from Dr. Kreipe. Dr. Slap invited her to interview with the program, indicating that they were interested in her strong eating disorder training from the University of Rochester. While Dr. Mitan and her family were not seeking career moves at the time, she decided to interview, and fell in love with the institution. She was recruited in 1999 to start an eating disorder presence, which would later become a formal program.

The program started slowly with a few referrals. Over twenty years later, there is now a large multidisciplinary team of clinicians, mental health providers, dietitians, and nurse care managers devoting sixty clinical hours per week to exclusively seeing patients who have eating disorders. Dr. Mitan became the program's first medical director in 2008. In the program's twenty years, there has been nearly an eightfold increase in the number of patients. In addition to leading this interdisciplinary ambulatory program, she also oversees the hospital's robust inpatient service, which provides medical stabilization to patients who have severe malnutrition. In 2012, she received a philanthropic gift earmarked for programmatic support and growth. As a result of the gift, Dr. Mitan was able to recruit a psychologist interested in eating disorders. They were then able to create a specific eating disorder fellowship with a psychology track, from which they were able to hire graduates of that program. "We've grown the program by literally starting at the grass roots level of having no providers to then hiring people who then trained more people whom we then hired," she said. It was a highly productive strategy recruiting clinicians and researchers, which most recently eventuated in the program receiving its first National Institutes of Health (NIH) grant in 2020, a major milestone in the history of the program.

Rightfully so, this program development is one of Dr. Mitan's proudest accomplishments in her career. "It's no longer built on just the hard work of one person, but it's truly a stand-alone, financially viable, well-respected program in our community," she said. However, what she remains most proud of is the relationships she has built with her patients and families throughout the years, evidenced through the wedding invitations, photographs of college graduations, and other souvenirs of her patients' milestone moments that she has received.

Dr. Mitan has witnessed many changes in the field throughout her career, perhaps most notably that adolescent medicine has become a more integral part of pediatric and family medicine care. "I feel like our society, our inner circle of adolescent medicine-trained people, don't have to work so hard for other people to understand what we do," she said with a laugh. She remembers having to explain the field to colleagues at national meetings, but now Dr. Mitan sees general pediatricians providing "a higher level and depth of adolescent care," including mental health and gynecological care. "I really credit adolescent medicine colleagues with getting that word out," she said. She has also seen an increase in the number of family medicine trained residents applying for fellowship. "I think adolescent medicine now has a strong foothold in all of the residency programs, not just pediatrics," she said. "It's broader, it's more core accepted, and it's obviously improving the outcomes of adolescents because we are reaching more of them."

Dr. Mitan has experienced success throughout her career and has contributed greatly to the field of adolescent medicine. Through her innovative programmatic development, strong relationships with patients and families, and educational efforts, the communities she has served have greatly benefited from her leadership and compassionate care. Her leadership is appreciated both inside and outside the Cincinnati area extending through her research, training the next generation of providers of care for adolescents, and outstanding clinical care of adolescents who have eating disorders and their families. An interest became a dream and gradually, over two decades, a reality.

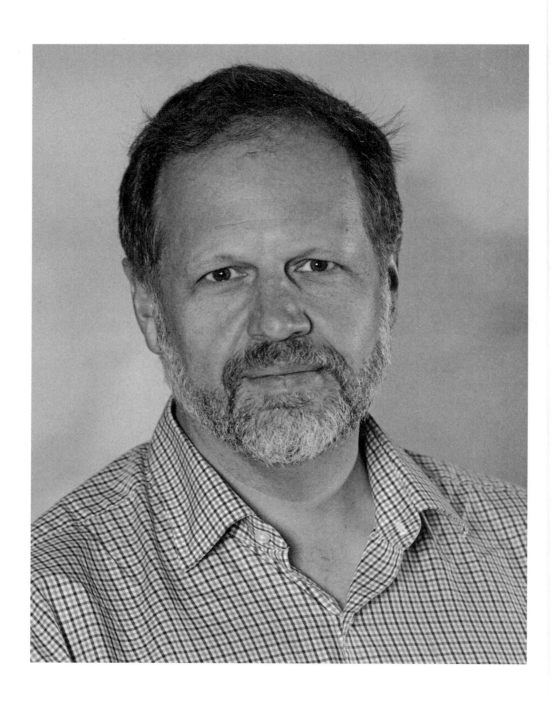

Chapter Seventeen

STEVE NORTH, MD, MPH, FAAFP

Steve North has devoted his career to caring for families and improving access to care, becoming a national leader in telehealth. With residency training in family medicine, Dr. North brought a unique perspective to the University of Rochester's Adolescent Medicine Fellowship program when he was a fellow from 2004 to 2006. His passions for education, school-based health, rural health, and adolescent and family medicine have seamlessly merged through the creation of a nonprofit organization, Health e-Schools, which is a national model for using telehealth in schools, and is improving access to healthcare for students in rural North Carolina.

North grew up in Wausau, Wisconsin, in a science-focused family. His mother was a clinical instructor in anatomy, physiology, and biochemistry and his father was a family physician. "My dad was an amazing doctor who practiced in our community for 35+ years," Dr. North said. "He talked to his patients at the grocery store and in front of our church on Sunday. He knew their stories and knew who they were." His father was an active member of the University of Wisconsin's Department of Family Medicine, founded a family medicine residency program, and started a hospice program in their community. Witnessing his father's work and the relationships he formed with those for whom he cared left a significant imprint on Steve.

North attended the University of Wisconsin-Madison for his undergraduate degree, where he pursued multiple educational interests. During his junior year, he learned about Teach for America (TFA), a program that placed college graduates in areas where there were teacher shortages, and found it aligned with his interests. After receiving acceptances to both medical school and the TFA program, he ultimately chose TFA and was placed in rural eastern North Carolina. He taught exceptional education in a grade 3–8 school, and though it was challenging, it was also rewarding. It was during this time that he was given a book about school-based health centers (SBHCs), of which there were approximately thirty across the country at the time. "It helped me see where medicine and education intersected, and it was amazing," he said. "It really changed what I wanted to do." He realized the immense power SBHCs could have on rural communities, witnessing firsthand the living conditions of many of his students. "I had kids who lived in shotgun shacks, who had cold water taps in the house and outhouses," he said, noting this was not uncommon in the rural south. After two years of teaching, he moved to Chapel Hill, North Carolina, where he pursued work in public health and rural medicine in preparation for medical school.

North attended medical school at the University of North Carolina at Chapel Hill with a goal of pursuing family medicine. "It was clear to me that I wanted to be a family doctor because I wanted to serve communities. I had seen my dad do it," he said. "I knew the way to really affect change for a family was to look at the whole family system." After marrying one of his medical school classmates, the couple moved to Rochester, New York, to begin their residency training at the University of Rochester.

Dr. North's interest in SBHCs persisted, and Rochester served as an excellent training ground, as there were several throughout the city. His involvement began quite serendipitously, as he lived in Rochester near Highland Hospital, the site of the Family Medicine residency program, which was across the street from School 12. While voting in the 2000 elections at School 12, medical assistance was needed for a staff member and Dr. North was able to help. This encounter opened a door for Dr. North to be involved in the school, where he ultimately developed a rotation for family medicine residents. "It wasn't to practice medicine, but to learn what kids experience at school because for many of us, we hadn't been in a public school since we were there as students," he said. "What does an Individualized Education Plan (IEP) look like? What are the things that kids are facing?" He met Dr. David

Broadbent, a pediatric leader in Rochester who was instrumental in the creation and management of SBHCs within the Rochester City School District, which served thousands of students. Through this relationship, his education and interest in SBHCs continued to grow.

While in residency, he also received external funding to create the Rochester Summer Health Externship Program, which allowed five high school students to rotate through multiple departments at the University of Rochester's affiliated Highland Hospital, providing experiences and exposure to youth who would not otherwise have that opportunity. Dr. North remains proud of that program and has kept in touch with several of the students, who went on to have careers in healthcare, psychology, and education. He remained at the Family Medicine residency for a chief year and then, still finding himself passionate about SBHCs, joined the Adolescent Medicine Fellowship program and concomitant Leadership Education in Adolescent Health (LEAH) program.

Dr. North was exposed to all aspects of adolescent medicine and particularly enjoyed the complex patients for whom he cared on the inpatient unit, as well as his experiences in the community at the Anthony Jordan Health Center and various SBHCs. Above all, he enjoyed his experiences teaching and engaging with the medical students. "That was really an amazing part for me," he said. In fact, something he remains most proud of is receiving the annual teaching award given by medical students.

Dr. North brought unique, important contributions to the fellowship as the program's first family medicine-trained physician. "I think my background in family medicine and my experience with seeing long-term complications of what happened during childhood in the clinical setting just gave me a different way to engage," he said. "I was able to provide a different perspective on family systems, and I think I brought the ability to look at transitions of care a little bit differently." Rochester's Division of Adolescent Medicine shared in his outlook on the importance of family. He can remember discussing a patient with Dr. Elizabeth McAnarney, who replied, "You know, Steve, it really is all about the family." He recalls, "That made me feel like I fit in even though I was not a pediatrician," he said.

Upon his fellowship graduation, Dr. North and his wife moved back to her hometown, Spruce Pine, in the Blue Ridge Mountains of Western North Carolina. Steve returned to join the Bakersville Community Medical Clinic, a rural health center in a town of 300, where he had done his third-year family medicine rotation. In 1996, they had founded two School and Family Health Centers (SFHCs), satellite clinics at rural schools, in the Buladean and Tipton Hill communities. The SFHCs had stopped being clinic locations and were providing only nursing care. Steve thought, "Rural schools are the hub of the community, so how do we increase engagement? By bringing people as patients there." He secured grant funding and was able to relaunch the centers as clinic sites that he staffed, creating the model of community clinics in schools that he envisioned while he was teaching. Unfortunately, in 2012 both schools and health centers closed due to declining attendance.

In 2007, with a desire to expand access to health care for rural students, Dr. North pursued the Jim Bernstein Community Health Leaders Fellowship, a program created in honor of Jim Bernstein, creator of Area Health Education Centers (AHECs) in the mid-1970s and secretary for the Department of Health and Human Services in North Carolina. Leadership fellows were selected based on their ideas for community health improvement. Dr. North's insights came from interactions he had in Rochester with Department of Pediatrics faculty, Drs. Neil Herendeen and Kenneth McConnochie, who had built a school-based telehealth program. Dr. North realized the impact telemedicine could have in reaching students at rural schools. He was accepted into the program and developed a needs assessment. "One of the great things was I received my Masters in Public Health (MPH) in Rochester, which provided both research skills and community development skills," he said. In 2011, after receiving several grants, he formed a nonprofit organization, the Center for Rural Health Innovation (CRHI), with the support of multiple local community members. After four years of research, program design, and fundraising, CRHI launched the Health-e-Schools program as a three-school pilot project for school-based telemedicine. They saw seventy-five students in the first year and have since grown to become a nationally recognized model providing care in 115 schools across nine counties in North Carolina. Additionally, CRHI provides telehealth care at a county jail and at two rural community centers, including Tipton Hill, the former site of a center. "We are now the largest independent school-based telemedicine program in the country," he said.

Health-e-Schools employs physicians and family nurse practitioners who see patients virtually while a trained presenter is on-site at the school with the student. The presenter is most often the school nurse, however front office staff, physical education teachers, and fire responders also present patients to the doctors and nurses. Advancements in technology resulting in lower prices have allowed for the program's expansion. Currently, clinical information obtained through stethoscopes and otoscopes can be transmitted to iPads via a portable handheld device. "We're watching everything that happens, and it runs like a regular school-based health center otherwise," Dr. North explained. In addition to improving access to care for all community members, they have seen significant impact on youth education. "These are Health Policy Shortage Areas, and it has really made a difference in keeping kids in schools," he said. Over 90% of students return to class after their visit. Prior to Health-e-Schools the majority of these students would have left school early and missed at least a half a day, having an impact on both their learning and the ability of their family members to go to work.

When reflecting on his career, the Health-e-Schools school-based telemedicine program is among his proudest accomplishments. "But I'm also proud of the fact that I'm a physician who has been here for fifteen years and families know me," he said. "At one point I took care of five generations of the same family." Being part of the community has brought him much fulfillment, and he comments on seeing patients at the grocery store and watching children grow up—connections that are amplified in a small community where everyone knows one another, and similar to situations that he witnessed his father encounter years ago.

While his family practice has gone beyond the scope of adolescents, he has certainly still cared for this population and has witnessed growth, new challenges, and opportunities in the field. "Autonomy for adolescents has become much more the focus. Privacy, confidentiality, but also supporting adolescents in a way that they can make their own decisions and giving that power, helping them understand their health," he said. "But at the same time, that has been in siloes in adolescent medicine and it's hard to see pediatric and family medicine practices who do not understand confidentiality." He has seen the field play an important and significant role in gender affirming care, an area he believes will continue to grow. However, he also worries about a future potential divide in the care that will be allowed to be delivered based on geographic area and associated legislation. Dr. North serves on the board of Advocates for Youth, an advocacy and education organization focused on adolescent and young adult sexual health rights, equity, accessibility, and confidentiality. He has seen success in reaching a marginalized population but hopes that youth who do not appear to be outwardly struggling are not missed, which he says will require accessibility to specialty adolescent healthcare outside of academia and within the primary care system. "I think telehealth is going to help a lot with that," he said.

Throughout his career, Dr. North has become a national expert in telemedicine. He has coauthored position papers for the American Telemedicine Association, one of which was adopted as the American Academy of Pediatrics' guideline for telemedicine in 2016, has served on national telehealth committees, and has become a go-to reviewer for matters involving adolescence and telemedicine. His commitment to caring for families, advocating for equitable healthcare, and substantially improving access to care in rural areas, has caused great improvements within the communities he serves and beyond. His nationally recognized telehealth model and expertise has expanded the way care is offered and obtained and has utilized our digital era to improve healthcare access and equity.

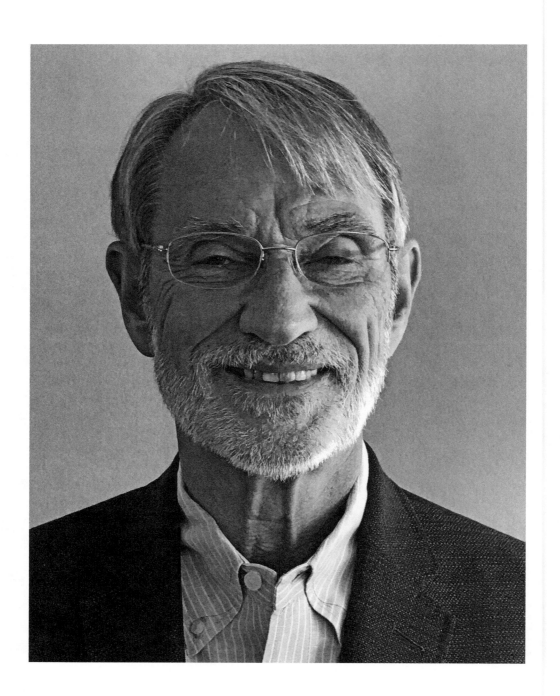

Chapter Eighteen

DONALD P. ORR, MD

Donald Orr graduated from the combined fellowship programs in General Academic Pediatrics and Child Psychiatry at the University of Rochester in 1976, following which he served on the Division of Adolescent Medicine faculty. Having spent the majority of his career as the founding director of Adolescent Medicine at Indiana University School of Medicine (IUSM), his leadership has made a great impact on the field on local, national, and international levels. His dedication to and ability to weave a strong research base into all clinical missions led to the creation of successful programs and important advances in knowledge related to adolescence. Dr. Orr officially retired in 2009, but his legacy continues to live on through IU's Dr. Donald P. Orr endowment, a true testament to the advancements he has made both clinically and through research.

Orr grew up in Orrville, Ohio, a small town founded by and named after his ancestors. As a young man, he was passionate about both music and science, and had some exposure to the medical world through his father, who was a pharmacist. He attended Ohio State University for his undergraduate education and originally pursued dental school after his first two years of college. However, after one quarter, it became clear to him that dentistry was not his perfect fit, so he finished his undergraduate education and went on to pursue medicine and receive his medical degree from Case Western Reserve School of Medicine in 1970.

He remembers having a unique medical school experience with an introduction to clinical medicine beginning the very first week, as well as a significant exposure to research through a required research dissertation. "I gave my first platform presentation at a national scientific meeting as a medical student," he said. "I was terrified, but it set me into the idea that research was important." His first clinical rotation was pediatrics, and on that rotation, he had an influential mentor who emphasized the importance of going onto the inpatient units and talking with children and their parents. At the time, Cleveland had one of the largest cystic fibrosis centers, so Orr found himself talking to many adolescents who had the disease, which he believes played a large role in determining his career. "I liked talking to adolescents and taking care of them," he said.

He remained in Cleveland for his pediatric residency. While he was determined to pursue adolescent medicine, he had taken his pediatric boards after his first year of residency (an early option that was allowed at the time), and found that there were not any adolescent medicine fellowship programs that would accept someone without first completing a three-year pediatrics residency. Thus, he applied for grant funding through the National Cystic Fibrosis Research Foundation to complete a one-year clinical fellowship in Pediatric Pulmonology and Adolescent Medicine at the University of Colorado Medical Center in Denver, which he accomplished before being enlisted to the Navy under the Berry Plan.

While stationed at Camp Pendleton in California, he cared for some teenagers and served as a consultant to the Adolescent Clinic, which made it clear to him that he was still interested in adolescent medicine, as well as equally evident that he was *not* interested in a purely clinical career. He longed for a research component, so before he was discharged from the Navy, he looked for opportunities in research training. Ironically, he turned down a faculty position from Dr. Morris Green, then chair of Pediatrics at Indiana University's Riley Hospital for Children, and created a plan to complete a research fellowship with Dr. I. Barry Pless, who was an investigator with the Rochester Child Health Study at the University of Rochester (UR). Right before Dr. Orr arrived, however, Dr. Pless left the UR. Since Dr. Orr's wife had accepted a faculty position in the Department of Psychology, they maintained their move to Rochester. Dr. Orr arranged for a fellowship with Dr. Robert Hoekelman, then head of Ambulatory Pediatrics and later chair of Pediatrics, to spend one-half of his time in Pediatrics and one-half in Child Psychiatry.

Much of his fellowship was spent working on a follow-up to the Child Health Study with children who were now teenagers, while also spending time each week in the adolescent medicine clinic. Dr. Orr remembers Rochester Adolescent Medicine as a strong program and one of the oldest programs in the field, one that has remained strong over time. Upon his graduation, he joined the Adolescent Medicine faculty, led by Dr. Elizabeth McAnarney, for a short time before going to the University of California at Irvine in their newly created medical school. He spent five years there before he went to IUSM to start an Adolescent Medicine Division. "I had decided when I had moved that anything we did clinically would have research embedded into it," he said, and he utilized his Robert Wood Johnson grant to create partnerships in the community. He started an on-site mental health program for middle school adolescents and credits a "very cooperative school board" with letting him collect data each year from the students by questionnaire that focused on health and sexual behaviors. He and his team were able to follow the seventh-grade students for four years. This project was the very first longitudinal study of adolescent sexual behavior and health behaviors in the United States.

Additionally, during his time establishing and leading IU's Division of Adolescent Medicine, he began a transitional clinic for teenagers who had diabetes, which also included a research component and received funding from the Centers for Disease Control (CDC), Maternal and Child Health Bureau (MCHB), and the National Institutes of Health (NIH) for diabetes and behavioral research. In 1991, IU became one of the seven programs for interdisciplinary training in adolescent health funded by the Department of Health and Human Services (DHHS) Maternal and Child Health Division. This allowed interdisciplinary faculty in medicine, nutrition, social work, and psychology to be hired. He also maintained a sexually transmitted infections (STIs) research clinical center for adolescents, which received continuous funding throughout his thirty-year tenure. He led two large, longitudinal studies that followed a cohort of 300 teenagers over eight years, collecting data that allowed them to link daily behavioral data to biologic outcomes.

At the time of his retirement in 2009, the division had grown to include eight physicians, four PhD investigators, and thirty staff. Building a strong division, which has remained strong after his departure, is among the accomplishments of which he is most proud in his career, including the solid research component he embedded into all clinical missions. "I think that our research with both diabetes and with STIs helped researchers, and eventually clinicians, understand adolescent behavior," he said, explaining that they found adolescent judgment and behavior are not as erratic and risk-taking as many believe.

His legacy is carried on within IU Adolescent Medicine through a Dr. Donald P. Orr Endowed Professorship and endowment. It was also in 2009 that he received the Outstanding Achievement in Adolescent Medicine award from the Society for Adolescent Health and Medicine (SAHM), a lifetime achievement award given to individuals nationally and internationally in recognition of their commitment to improving the health of adolescents and young adults.

Reflecting on the progress in the field, Dr. Orr says, "Adolescent medicine as a field within academics is solid. It is going to continue. It's embedded in all Departments of Pediatrics and there are more pediatricians now, who are the mainstay of child healthcare, who are being trained to take care of adolescents in a meaningful way." He believes one of the biggest challenges is to "find ways to promote research at the fellow level for those who strongly want to pick that up as a challenge." However, he has seen improvement in the research experience adolescent medicine fellows receive, which is something he had to seek out and build for himself, learning as he went. "I think one of the big advances in adolescent medicine fellowships is that there is a research requirement," he said.

Dr. Orr has accomplished much throughout his career, including serving as the leader of a large multi-disciplinary Adolescent Medicine division, an esteemed researcher, an associate editor for national journals, including *Journal of Adolescent Health* and *Diabetes Care,* and a subject matter expert who has served as an advisor and consultant on many national committees and initiatives related to adolescent health. His dedication and tireless efforts to improve care and knowledge around important adolescent issues has improved understanding and positively affected the health of countless adolescents. Dr. Orr's legacy in adolescent medicine is strong and highly meaningful.

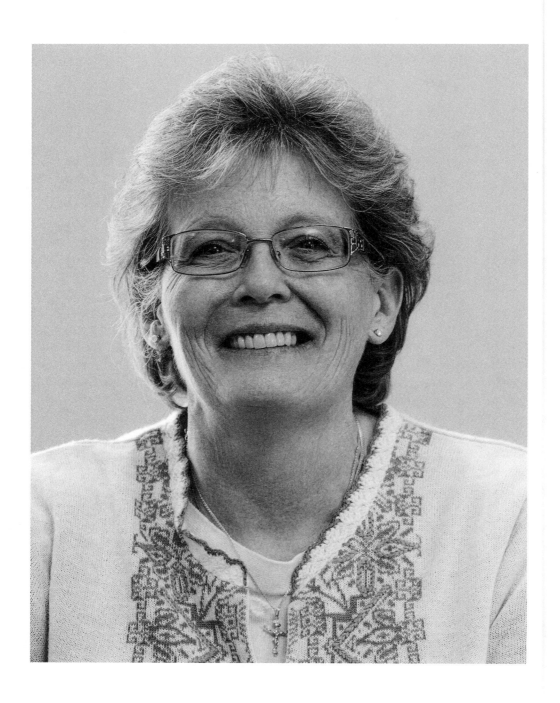

Chapter Nineteen

KATHY H. RIDEOUT, EdD, PPCNP-BC, FNAP

Kathy Rideout has had an esteemed nursing career, which includes serving as dean of the University of Rochester (UR) School of Nursing for ten years. In her early days as a nurse practitioner, she worked closely with the Division of Adolescent Medicine, a group that she says truly valued and emphasized multidisciplinary care and created an environment that was instrumental in her development as a nursing leader.

Rideout grew up in Pittsburgh, Pennsylvania, the youngest of five girls. Her mother was a nurse's aide and would often talk about how much she loved her job, her patients, and working in the hospital. Rideout began volunteering as a "candy-striper" during her early high school years, which solidified her decision to pursue nursing. During that time, there was a greater emphasis than previously on obtaining a baccalaureate degree in nursing from a four-year program, as opposed to receiving a three-year diploma or a two-year associate degree, which had been the standard. She attended Indiana University of Pennsylvania (IUP) and worked as a nurse's aide in the same hospital as her mother during her summer breaks from college. Upon graduating with her Bachelor of Science in Nursing (BSN), she began working at Children's Hospital of Pittsburgh before moving to a smaller hospital closer to home to avoid the high costs of the commute.

During this time in the early 1980s, the role of the nurse practitioner was starting to evolve, which interested Dr. Rideout greatly. She attended the University of Pittsburgh for her master's degree as a pediatric nurse practitioner (PNP) and clinical nurse specialist, graduating in 1983. While working in

Pittsburgh, she met her husband, whose career moved the couple to Rochester. "The only thing I knew about Rochester was Dr. Lee Ford, the first dean of the UR School of Nursing," she said. "She founded the PNP role and model of education, so I knew that the University of Rochester was really where I wanted to be." Thus, she interviewed and was offered a position that involved teaching and working at Golisano Children's Hospital, which at the time in 1986, was called the Children's Hospital at Strong and was comprised of four units on a single floor, one of which was the adolescent unit—a unit on which Dr. Rideout played an integral role for eighteen years. It was during this time that she worked with Dr. Elizabeth McAnarney, who was the Adolescent Medicine division chief, and the other adolescent medicine faculty members, including Dr. Richard Kreipe. "They really valued interprofessional care, which was very important to me," she said. "We always sat down as a team of nurses, social workers, child life specialists, adolescent medicine attendings, fellows, and residents—it was really a team approach in anything we did."

With a love for teaching and a drive to advance her career, Dr. Rideout pursued her doctorate degree at the UR's Warner School of Education and Human Development. She completed a postdoctoral fellowship with pediatric clinician-researcher, Harriet Kitzman, PhD, RN, in which they studied different collaborative care models on the adolescent unit. "We felt that it was important for there to be a continuity of care that couldn't happen with residents and fellows because they rotated all the time," she said. Thus, she developed a model in which a nurse practitioner (NP) served as care coordinator for a select group of patients on the unit, specifically focusing on patients who had eating disorders and/or cystic fibrosis, as both groups had frequent readmissions. In this model, the NP care coordinator was alerted when a patient was going to be admitted so that the appropriate services such as nutrition or pulmonary care were in place and the team was ready at the time of admission. After utilizing this model, they found an increase in efficiency of services provided, a decrease in length of stay, and ultimately, improved patient satisfaction due to the continuity of care. While this concept of NP care coordination is more routine now, with over 800 nurse practitioners currently working in the institution, it was novel during this time when the nurse practitioner role in acute care was still fairly new and there were not many practicing in acute care environments. Dr. Rideout served in this care coordinator role for two years during her postdoctoral fellowship and said she could not have done it without the support of the Division of Adolescent Medicine. "That was just how they provided care—in a team approach. It wasn't threatening that there was an actual nurse practitioner that was part of the team coordinating the inpatient care; they really saw it as an added benefit for the care of patients on the unit."

One of her proudest accomplishments is helping embed the importance of interprofessional and collaborative care. "No matter how busy the adolescent unit was, we always had times where we sat down as a team and really looked at what are all the factors contributing to either the physical issues an adolescent was experiencing, or the behavioral mental health issues," she said. "And everything we did was based on an interprofessional model—it was just second nature for us. Nurses did not make their own decisions, medicine did not make their own decisions, and social work did not make their own decisions. We really did that as a team." She credits Drs. McAnarney and Kreipe for setting that stage and promoting that philosophy of care.

After receiving her doctorate, she became the director of the PNP program at the School of Nursing, while still maintaining a clinical role in the hospital. When Dr. Walter Pegoli became the chief of Pediatric Surgery, he wanted to hire an ostomy nurse specialist and Dr. Rideout expressed interest. She feels fortunate she had the opportunity to go back to school and become an ostomy specialist, specializing in the care of infants, children, and adolescents. When she moved to the associate dean position and then later to dean, she was able to maintain her role as ostomy nurse, placing her in the hospital each day, which she says is extremely helpful. In fact, this is the role she remains most proud of in her career—"The fact that I've never let go of the importance of still practicing as a nurse"—noting that it is unique for a dean to continue to practice clinically. "When I was offered the associate dean position, I said I would only do so if I could continue to practice because that's who I am—I am a nurse and it really informs everything I do." When she subsequently accepted the position of dean, she once again had it written in her contact that she would still be able to practice. "I garner so much satisfaction in being a nurse," she said. "It still gives me that connection to patients and our families and to providers. And so I think I'm really most proud of the fact that I've been able to continue to do that."

When Dr. Rideout was named dean of the School of Nursing in 2012, she asked Dr. McAnarney to speak at her installation. "I really saw her as a key part of my professional development," she said. "NP roles hadn't evolved that much and so to come into an environment where nursing was so respected and there was an openness to look at different roles and different ways of doing things and really having that team approach ... to grow up in that environment was very instrumental in my development as a nursing leader."

Dr. Rideout said her time working with the Division of Adolescent Medicine provided her with many skills and lessons that have influenced her success as dean. She learned the importance of having a trusted mentor—"You can't lead by yourself without guidance or advice from someone wiser than yourself"—and the importance of having a sense of humor—"Sometimes when we take life events too seriously, it can be crippling." She learned to view every crisis as a season: "There are changes that are happening constantly and how you view the situation and help others view the situation are critical. Reframing the 'crisis' can help inform how we manage the situation successfully." She learned to understand that not everything you do or try will be successful: "Rethinking, reorganizing, re-strategizing are the foundations for success—it does not mean you have failed." Further, she gained appreciation that everyone's point of view is valuable: "We all have a different lens and appreciating each other's lens is critical to either providing the best care, the best solutions to a problem or in the development of new initiatives."

Throughout her career, she has witnessed the important role of adolescent medicine. "It is such a critical time in development. There's a whole different way that you approach an adolescent with a chronic or an acute illness than you do, obviously, with a toddler or preschooler," she said, noting the importance of having the understanding about how critical that time period is, particularly surrounding mental health. "I think the history of adolescent medicine of paying attention to those issues many, many decades ago has really helped inform the care that kids receive now," she said. "They were paying attention to it long before anyone else was paying attention to it. Now I think it's taken for granted that of course we pay attention to the behavioral and mental health issues of teenagers, but that was embedded decades ago." Additionally, she notes the importance of a specialty that views the whole child, taking into account complex family and behavioral issues that often transcend the medical diagnosis. "Having that specialty to be able to peel away the onion and look at what is the significance of the mental health issues and the developmental issues that are impacting a teenager—diagnosed, for example, with Crohn's disease, diabetes, or cancer—is critical," she said. She can vividly remember being a part of that interprofessional team, sitting around the table in the back room, discussing the whole child. She said she will run into former team members from time to time and they will all agree, "Those were the best days of our lives."

The collaborative care and respect she felt as an NP on the adolescent unit is something she said is easy to take for granted, as it is the environment in which she "grew up." She feels fortunate to have had that experience, one that she also feels at the university level, noting the genuine partnership she has with the senior leaders of the institution, which is something her nursing school dean counterparts at other institutions admire greatly. "I couldn't imagine working in an environment where that wasn't the case, and I think we need to recognize how special that is," she said.

In her role as the dean of the School of Nursing, Dr. Rideout has exemplified compassionate, informed, and energetic role modelling. She and her colleagues at the school have attracted hundreds of students of all backgrounds and ages to emulate the great traditions of the leaders of the nursing profession, such as Dr. Rideout. The adolescents she has served and is serving clinically and the students, faculty, and the UR Medical Center staff whom she leads have all benefited immensely from her leadership.

Dean Rideout's thoughtful and informed leadership has not only contributed to the remarkable and positive changes during her ten-year term as dean, but has also benefited the URMC and the profession of nursing locally and nationally. Dr. Rideout has left an indelible mark on each area in which she worked. Ultimately, it is Dr. Rideout's patients, families, and trainees who will remember most vividly her great influence.

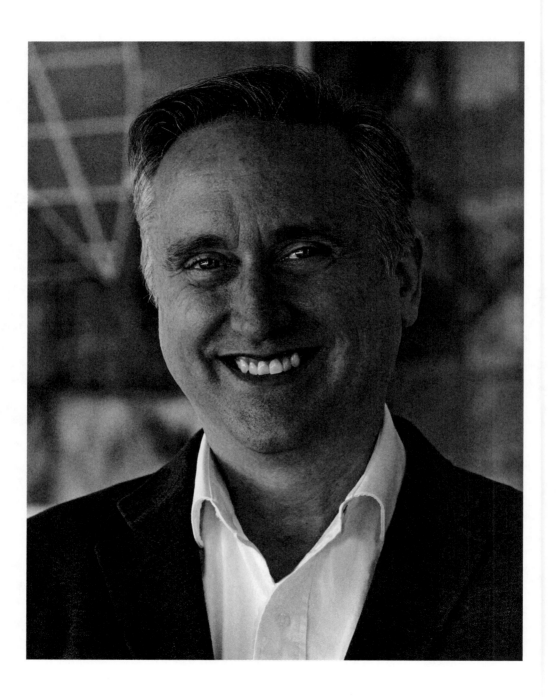

Chapter Twenty

BRETT W. ROBBINS, MD

Brett Robbins has devoted much of his career to medical education as the internal medicine–pediatrics residency program director, vice chair for education in the Department of Medicine, and the Graduate Medical Education (GME) assistant designated institutional official (DIO) for medical specialties at the University of Rochester School of Medicine and Dentistry (URSMD). He is a graduate of the URSMD internal medicine–pediatrics residency program and is now professor of Medicine and Pediatrics. However, he also has an important role in the history of Rochester's Adolescent Medicine program, as he served as division chief from 2009 to 2017. One of his strengths and core interests is to help develop young physicians in their careers—whether that be at the resident, fellow, or faculty level—and is something he contributed to greatly during his tenure as division chief.

Robbins grew up in northern Indiana in a small suburb outside of Chicago, and according to his mother, he had aspirations of becoming a physician beginning at the young age of four years old. He attended a small liberal arts university, Hanover College, for his undergraduate education, followed by Indiana University School of Medicine. Throughout his medical education, he realized medicine *and* pediatrics made him the happiest and feels fortunate to have matched at the University of Rochester's combined internal medicine–pediatrics residency program, which he completed from 1993 to 1997. He fondly remembers that Dr. Elizabeth McAnarney was one of his first attending physicians on the adolescent medicine unit. Although his original plan was to return to Indiana following residency to become a primary care physician, he says, "I fell in love with the learning environment in Rochester, which I define as genuine and psychologically safe. The real tenet of that, which I was taught and now teach others, is to embrace what you don't know and not fear it," which he says is not always the case at institutions of higher learning. "It never made sense to me to make people feel bad if they didn't already know something they had yet to learn," he said.

Dr. Robbins eagerly joined the faculty at the University of Rochester upon his graduation, primarily spending time at Rochester General Hospital (RGH) as an ambulatory preceptor in the ambulatory medicine-pediatrics practice and as an inpatient general medicine hospitalist. In his first year after residency, Dr. Lynn Garfunkel, who was serving as interim program director for the URSMD internal medicine–pediatrics residency, appointed Dr. Robbins as associate program director. In a short two years later, he assumed the role of program director. He enthusiastically accepted, but asked to be sent to a Health Resources and Services Administration (HRSA)–funded one-year faculty development fellowship at Michigan State University. He would often consider for which specialty he would pursue fellowship training, but said, "In my heart-of-hearts I am a generalist, and the only things that would come to mind were things where I could still be a generalist. I just couldn't focus on one organ or one system." Thus, he was grateful for the faculty development experience he received at Michigan State. He has now served as program director for over twenty years—a role that has brought him much fulfillment, joy, and pride.

In 2009, during his tenth year as program director, he received a phone call from the then chair of the Department of Pediatrics, Dr. Nina Schor, who asked Dr. Robbins to step in as interim chief of the Division of Adolescent Medicine. There was a formal recruitment process underway, so the assignment was projected to be a six-month duration. "I said sure—I didn't have a fellowship [in adolescent medicine], but I could hopefully hold things together for six months," he said with a laugh. He dove right in by joining the Society for Adolescent Health and Medicine (SAHM), studying the field's national landscape, and learning the team and each person's interests and career goals, as well as learning about the three-year adolescent medicine fellowship program. "It was quite the steep learning curve," he said. Over time, Dr. Robbins decided to apply for the permanent position—"mostly because I fell in love with the team that we had there," he said. Thus, what began as a six-month interim assignment turned into eight wonderful years for Dr. Robbins and for the Division of Adolescent Medicine.

He remembers those years as a turning point for the division. Previously, there had been a major focus on adolescent eating disorders, which former division chief, Dr. Richard Kreipe, helped bring to the forefront through his internationally renowned scholarly and clinical work in the field. Dr. Kreipe's leadership brought national recognition to Rochester's eating disorder program, which continues to be prominent today. When Dr. Robbins began his tenure, adolescent eating disorders remained a strong focus of the program. Additionally, there were several young women physicians who had slightly different career aspirations. While they wanted to keep eating disorders as a major component, they also had visions of expanding services in reproductive health. Dr. Robbins helped facilitate their vision by working to collaborate and align the division with the Department of Obstetrics and Gynecology, orchestrating new contracts, equipment, and training, as well as modifying templates for scheduling, patient appointments, and new counseling. "There were so many moving parts to our clinical mission at that point," he said. What was remarkable to him were the energy and passion each of these faculty members had, and the quickness with which they were able to achieve success from the ambitious goals they set for themselves. "There was never any shortage of energy, never any shortage of talent or desire to just do good things," he said. Further, "the beauty is that the care of the patient with eating disorders wasn't dropped or lessened in any way, it was just added to." The group did not diminish any of that previous renowned work or care, they just added to it in different areas.

The ways in which Dr. Robbins was able to help the junior adolescent medicine faculty develop their particular niche and career is something of which he is justly proud. He says he was not perfect at it, but tried to recognize what each person needed, and then advocate and push for resources to enable it. He says throughout his career, he has tried to emulate Dr. McAnarney's strong mentorship and ability to develop people, citing her as one of the most influential people in his career, as he often finds himself asking 'What would Lissa do?' "Being a leader in my mind is actually much more about developing those in your charge, not yourself," he said. "It was never about me. I did this to make sure that they were able to do what they wanted and needed to do. And I guess that's of what I'm most proud—is what they've done." Throughout all of the changes that occurred, he is proud that they remained a team and weathered those changes together. "I feel really good about the fact that the division was able to do such an amazingly good job at pivoting and broadening the clinical focus, broadening the scholarly focus really quickly with the addition of some key faculty, and the fact that we were able to stay a team in doing that. That was probably the most important thing that happened to me during that entire period of time."

In 2016, Dr. Robbins was presented with two new opportunities, which were very much aligned with his interest and passion for medical education. The chair of the Department of Medicine (Dr. Paul Levy) asked him to become the Department's vice chair for education. Practically simultaneously Dr. Diane Hartmann, the senior associate dean for Graduate Medical Education and DIO, asked him to become an assistant DIO, a position that would oversee the university's medical specialty and subspecialty training programs in Medicine, Pediatrics, Family Medicine, Neurology, Psychiatry, and Physical Medicine and Rehabilitation. He was excited about these opportunities and knew he could not remain division chief while taking on these additional responsibilities. He also knew that eventually the Division of Adolescent Medicine would need a chief with credentials in the field. He laughs, remarking that all physicians tend to have impostor syndrome from time-to-time, but he felt it even more so by not having board certification in the field of the division he was leading. He had been having conversations with Dr. Susan (Shellie) Yussman about becoming the next chief, and thus when he stepped down, she became interim chief before fully taking over the role in 2019.

Dr. Robbins accepted both educational leadership roles in addition to remaining the internal medicine–pediatrics residency program director. These three roles give him a unique perspective—he says he has a micro-level view as a residency program director himself, a more macro-level view as a vice chair for education, and a "30,000-foot view" as an assistant DIO helping to provide oversight for nearly 850 trainees. "That has afforded me an amazing amount of insight," he said. "When you have all three of those perspectives, they inform each other. It is great fun; I've got to say, I'm living the dream."

Dr. Robbins is grateful for his time leading the Division of Adolescent Medicine and says he misses the team, with whom he will always have a special connection. He is pleased that he is once again able to work closely with adolescent medicine faculty member, Dr. Taylor Starr, whom he hired as an associate residency program director for the internal medicine–pediatrics program—something he said was a "no-brainer." He is also especially grateful for the mentorship he has received from Dr. McAnarney during his time as division chief as well as throughout his whole career. "Just her presence and the way she moves in the world are so inspiring," he said. Reflecting on his time in Adolescent Medicine, he says, "The thing that I was most impressed with was how people were leveraging what small amount of federal, state, and local funding there was out there with the true intent of improving teenagers' lives. For the adolescent medicine folks, it's really about making the world better and that has held so true." As for the future, he says it is bright because of the people in the field and their genuine embracing of their mission. "One of my main mantras is 'don't get in their way.' Their hearts and their motivations are so pure; the worst thing you can do as their leader is stand in their way."

Dr. Robbins is a talented and committed leader who has accomplished much in his career. He says it is truly a love of developing young trainees that has influenced his career aspirations and successes, both as a leader in medical education and his time as division chief. "That has always been my main motive," he said. "Because it's such fun, it is an amazing thing to have a team of smart, wonderful, kind human beings around you." That is exactly what he thinks of the adolescent medicine group with whom he had the opportunity to work, and it brings him great pride to see what they have accomplished both individually and as a team. "It has been so fun to watch them get promoted, famous and accomplished, and that's honestly what it was always about for me."

Robbins' leadership and facilitation of growth during his time as chief enabled the Division of Adolescent Medicine to broaden its clinical and scholarly missions, which not only greatly affected the faculty and their individual career development and trajectories, but also the care of adolescents and young adults in the Rochester community. Dr. Robbins is truly a "man for all seasons" with his remarkable success emanating from his generativity, that is, giving to the next generation selflessly as he role-models superb clinical skills, insightful teaching, high integrity, and kindness. His reach has extended to all levels of the university, its School of Medicine and Dentistry, and even the Rochester Red Wings, the city's minor league baseball team, where Dr. Robbins is a team physician.

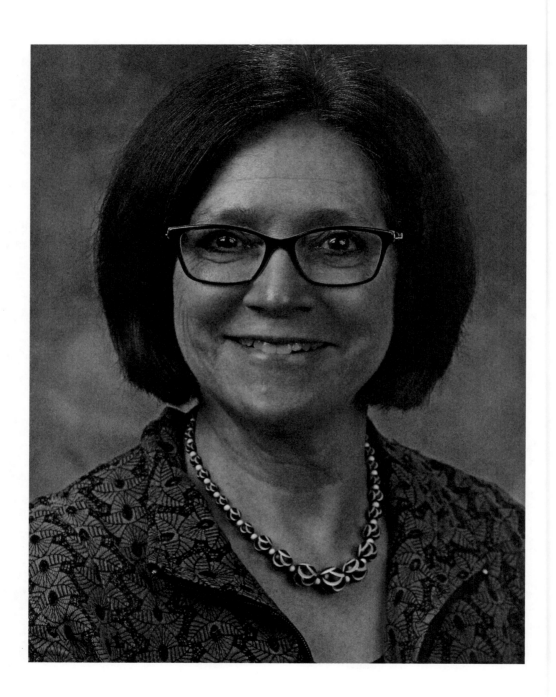

Chapter Twenty-One

Sheryl A. Ryan, MD

Sheryl Ryan has served as a leader, educator, and innovator in adolescent medicine throughout her career, including ten impactful years as a faculty member at the University of Rochester School of Medicine and Dentistry (URSMD) and its affiliated pediatrics program at Rochester General Hospital (RGH) from 1995 to 2005. She is professor of Pediatrics, division chief of Adolescent Medicine, and founder and program director of the interdisciplinary addiction medicine fellowship at Penn State Children's Hospital.

Ryan grew up in Massachusetts and attended Boston College for her undergraduate education, where she first aspired to be an early education teacher. She obtained a student teaching experience during her freshman year, and while it confirmed her interest in working with children, it was a visit to her pediatrician over the summer that piqued her interest in medicine. When she returned to Boston College, she applied to the School of Arts and Sciences and began catching up on premedical courses, something she was told would be an impossible feat as a sophomore. "When somebody tells me you can't do something, I'll make sure I can do it," she said. And that she did. She successfully changed course, was accepted into medical school, and chose to attend Yale School of Medicine. While she kept an open mind throughout each of her clinical rotations—all of which she enjoyed—her passion would always return to pediatrics.

She completed her residency in pediatrics at Children's Hospital of Philadelphia where her research interest in adolescent medicine developed. She was particularly interested in how adolescents utilized services in a way that was separate from their parents, as adolescence was a time when they were starting to make their own decisions regarding their medical needs and uses of services. It was this adolescent-focused research that led her to apply for a fellowship in adolescent medicine, which she completed at the University of California San Francisco (UCSF). Following fellowship, she returned to the East Coast for a postdoctoral fellowship in health services research at the Johns Hopkins Bloomberg School of Public Health. She remained in Baltimore for her first faculty position at the University of Maryland at Baltimore in the Division of Adolescent Medicine, which she held for five years before moving to Rochester, New York.

While it was her husband's career that brought the family to Rochester, it was an excellent fit for Dr. Ryan. She was well aware of the University of Rochester's strong program in adolescent medicine led by Dr. Elizabeth McAnarney, followed by Dr. Richard Kreipe. When she inquired about potential job possibilities, she was delighted to obtain a position with the university's affiliated pediatrics program at RGH. "It was an easy transition for me," she said, explaining that she was familiar with the Rochester group given the relatively small size of the field—a group with whom she was very excited to work. Although she was primarily located at RGH, she became very involved at the University of Rochester through teaching fellows and spending time clinically in both inpatient and outpatient settings.

Ryan also brought with her a unique experience and perspective that was instrumental in the Rochester Adolescent Medicine Program receiving its first Leadership Education in Adolescent Health (LEAH) grant in 1997. Having trained in a LEAH fellowship at UCSF and having served as the director of research for the University of Maryland's LEAH program, she was well-positioned to assist in applying for the competitive funding. "I was able to say, 'these are the components you need, let's bring them together,'" she said. "Everybody worked together extremely well."

Once funding was received, Ryan served as training director and was instrumental in helping create the multidisciplinary clinical experience, which brought together faculty and fellows from all five disciplines (nursing, nutrition, medicine, psychology, and social work) through a weekly clinic to collaborate on the care of complicated patients. A pair of fellows would see each patient while the faculty and remaining fellows observed through two-way mirrors. Throughout the visit, the group would convene, give real time feedback, and evaluate each patient and family together in a multidisciplinary fashion. "It was an incredibly rich learning opportunity because the fellows could hear what the professionals of all five disciplines said about the medical, social, and family issues," Ryan said. "And it was a great experience for the fellows to learn how to work with each other, which is what it was all about—interdisciplinary training. For me as a faculty member, it was one of the highlights of my week to be able to do this." Serving as the LEAH fellowship training director and mentoring fellows both clinically and in their scholarly work remain among Ryan's proudest contributions throughout her ten years on the University of Rochester faculty.

As her children reached the end of high school and were pursuing education in New England, and as her aging parents' medical needs necessitated Ryan's closer proximity to Massachusetts, she made the difficult decision to leave Rochester and accept a position at her medical school alma mater, Yale School of Medicine, as the division chief of Adolescent Medicine. It was a small division of one, which placed Ryan on call 24/7, 365 days of the year. She served in this role for twelve years. It was also during this time that she developed an interest in addiction through her work on the American Academy of Pediatrics (AAP) Committee for Substance Abuse. She served as the adolescent medicine physician tasked with developing the pediatric core around addiction medicine. "I began working with this great multi-department research group on developing education about addiction for pediatrics," she said. One of her committee coleaders was someone she trained with at UCSF who was chair of Pediatrics at Penn State College of Medicine. She recruited Ryan there to lead Penn State's large Adolescent Medicine Division of thirty-five people and to create a fellowship in addiction medicine.

Within her first year at Penn State, Ryan collaborated with six other departments and built the interdisciplinary fellowship in addiction medicine, which over the course of three years has received funding from a Health Resources and Services Administration (HRSA) grant and now supports four fellows. The fellowship is located in the Department of Pediatrics, but also includes members from the Departments of Internal Medicine, Emergency Medicine, Family Medicine, Obstetrics and Gynecology, Pain Medicine, and

Pharmacology, and recruits trainees from any primary care specialty. As Ryan went through the process of creating the fellowship, she said she drew from her experiences in Rochester. She has wonderful memories of working with colleagues on the LEAH didactic curriculum and recalled those experiences as she wrote the fellowship in addiction medicine, particularly the didactic component, which she modeled after the Rochester LEAH didactic curriculum. "With our LEAH grant, we were really able to involve the community and I think that informed me about just how rich and important the community involvement in teaching and training is," she said, noting that she has incorporated multiple community sites into her addiction medicine fellowship, something that applicants find unique. "We stand on the shoulders of great people. There are so many great colleagues I had when in Rochester, and that has informed what I'm doing now," she said. "I have a lot of people to thank for what I'm doing now."

Ryan is grateful for her experiences in Rochester, for those who served as mentors to her, including McAnarney and Kreipe, and for the fellows whom she was able to mentor and watch achieve great accomplishments in the field. "Rochester Adolescent Medicine has a very long tradition of really good, solid clinical care, as well as research," she said, noting the early work in positive youth development, and the Rochester Adolescent Maternity Program (RAMP) and Teen-Tot clinic, which were among the first of their kind. "They have been at the forefront of a lot; it has been a consistently great program that has had a lot of effect over many decades of pushing forward excellence in adolescent health." She is also grateful for the experiences and memories Rochester provided her family. Her children were just four and five years old when they moved to Rochester. "When we moved to New England in 2005, my daughter was starting college at Boston College and my son had just finished his sophomore year of high school. It was tough for them to move and they still will tell you that 'Rochester is where they grew up' and they have incredibly fond memories of their years there!" she said.

As for the future of adolescent health, the aftermath of the COVID-19 pandemic causes her to worry. She has witnessed firsthand the mental health crisis that has continued to plague adolescents, which she believes the pandemic has amplified. "COVID has highlighted the problems in the mental health system and the amount of stress and anxiety our young people are experiencing," she said. Further, "I think that society has created so much more anxiety and expectation for our young people, but at the same time, it's not protecting them from social media, the internet, and the kind of influences kids encounter. They are out there acquiring ideas but without a filter of adult experiences." The country's political climate is also worrisome to her, as she fears for the future of reproductive and gender health access, and adolescent consent and confidentiality. "And that is where we have to be advocates," she said. "We in adolescent medicine have to step up to the plate and advocate for our youth and young adults in ways that I didn't think we had to a couple of decades ago."

Dr. Ryan's contributions in adolescent health research, education, and mentorship have had a significant impact on the institutions and national organizations for which she has served and the trainees she has affected, and her leadership has been invaluable to the progress of the field.

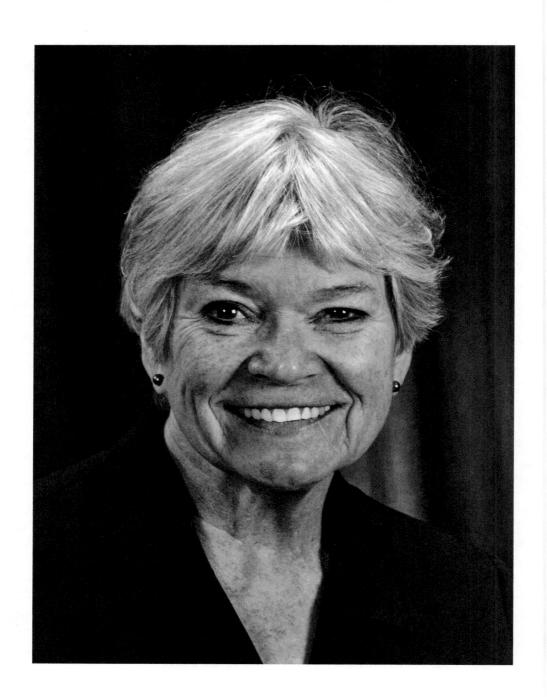

Chapter Twenty-Two

OLLE JANE (O.J.) SAHLER, MD

Olle Jane "O.J." Sahler identifies herself as a behavioral pediatrician, but has had a wonderfully diverse career taking care of adolescents as an esteemed member of the Division of Adolescent Medicine faculty, as well as in the Divisions of Hematology-Oncology, Palliative Care, and Medical Education. She has spent nearly all of her highly productive 50-year career at the University of Rochester Medical Center (URMC). As professor of Pediatrics, Psychiatry, Medical Humanities & Bioethics, and Oncology, she continues to play a fundamental role in the institution, Department of Pediatrics, and Division of Adolescent Medicine.

Growing up, Sahler has early memories of her father, a general practitioner turned ophthalmologist later in his career, using the front of their home as his office, waiting room, and treatment room. "It really made medicine a part of our family because it was always happening around us," she said, remembering local children coming to the back door with various injuries. However, regardless of that, she said her initial plan in life was to become a nun and a teaching missionary. That is, until her eighth-grade homeroom teacher challenged that idea and said, "You don't want to be a doctor like your father?" to which she replied, "Yeah, I want to be a doctor like my father!"

Her mind was made up, but her parents were not as enthusiastic. Her father saw firsthand the pressures that surrounded students while he was in medical school at Yale in the 1930s, as two students in his class, one of whom was a woman, committed suicide. He was therefore wary of his daughter pursuing a career in medicine. However, he was very supportive when she made the decision to attend the University of Rochester School of Medicine and

Dentistry (URSMD), home of the biopsychosocial model and an institution at which he had a wonderful experience interviewing for residency. He told her, "I really think you're going to find it to be a very special place." Sahler said she could feel that sense of caring at the University of Rochester that has always been a part of its legacy, and over fifty years later, she still finds it to be a very special place.

After graduation, Dr. Sahler and her husband, Dr. Carl "Chip" Sahler headed to Durham, North Carolina, for residencies at Duke University in pediatrics and internal medicine, respectively. This was part of a two-year deferment Dr. Chip Sahler received from the military, and when it came time for him to enlist, the Army was very interested in his wife's role as a pediatrician. If Dr. O.J. Sahler also joined, the couple could choose wherever they would like to go and they would not be separated. This was very important to them, for as an internist, Dr. Chip Sahler could have easily been sent to Vietnam. However, with the end of the war nearing and fewer people being deployed, a pediatrician's services were not needed there and they were able to head to California instead. While on base in Fort Ord, California, Dr. O.J. Sahler worked at Silas B. Hays Army Hospital and saw many young families during what were very difficult and unusual circumstances. These were young eighteen- to twenty-one-year-olds who were thousands of miles away from their families and were able to make a collect call home for only a few minutes each week. There was no opportunity for them to be nurtured and supported as they raised their own children, so they often turned to Dr. Sahler and her practice. It was a challenging and rewarding time in her career.

After the Sahlers' time in the Army ended, Dr. Chip Sahler was recruited back to the University of Rochester and Dr. O.J. Sahler contacted Dr. Elizabeth McAnarney, with whom she had worked as a medical student, about opportunities. With Dr. McAnarney's blessing, she was able to create a fellowship experience combining her varied interests in behavioral pediatrics, adolescent medicine, psychiatry, and family therapy, which she aptly named Behavioral/Developmental Pediatrics and Child & Adolescent Psychiatry. It was a hybrid experience that fit her needs perfectly. She had wonderful mentors as a medical student in Rochester, including the notable Drs. Stanford Friedman, George Engel, and John Romano, and looked forward to returning. Dr.

Friedman encouraged her to stay after fellowship and she was hired by Dr. David H. Smith, the fourth chair of the Department of Pediatrics.

She did not know it at the time, but Dr. Smith gave her an assignment that would have a huge impact on the trajectory of her career and would lead to one of her proudest contributions to the field of pediatrics. Dr. Smith appointed her as the pediatric clerkship director, the first female to hold this role in the institution, and gave her two directives: (1) make the clerkship your laboratory and (2) get involved in computer-assisted education. This was 1977 when the computers that were being used (48K Apples) had approximately the same storage size as the most simple text message in 2020. However, Sahler dove right in and was able to create a program called MEDCAPS (Medical Computer-Assisted Problem Solving) for the students to use.

She was also tasked with the ultimate goal of increasing the number of medical students who pursued pediatrics, which had most recently been four. When she reviewed the curriculum, she realized that the six-week exclusively inpatient experience was likely painting a grim picture for students, as during that time, therapies and treatments for cystic fibrosis, leukemia, and other childhood disorders were not what they would later be, and the hospital was oftentimes where these chronically ill children came to die. "Pediatrics back then, in the hospital, was a very sad affair," she said. Aiming to give students a fuller picture that included more positive outcomes, she made arrangements for them to rotate in clinics and practices in the community. This allowed them to see the patients who had cancer, but were going to survive, or those who had cystic fibrosis who were currently going to school and otherwise living normal lives. Within a period of two to three years, Dr. Sahler saw the number of students going into pediatrics triple and quadruple.

While she saw great success with this change in curriculum, she also remembers receiving much criticism from her all-male clerkship director colleagues in other departments—being told she was demeaning medical education and setting the bar too low. Keeping in line with Dr. Smith's first directive of making the clerkship her laboratory, she was inspired to seek out what pediatric clerkship directors at the 130 other schools around the country were doing and to compare practices. However, she quickly ran into an issue—such a list of directors did not exist. With a $300 grant from the Ambulatory

Pediatric Association (now the Academic Pediatric Association), she sent letters to pediatric department chairs across the country and began to compile a list, albeit very small at first. In 1985, she invited this small group to one of the spring scientific meetings held in California, reserved a conference room, and promised water! About twelve colleagues came, and that was the very beginning of the formation of the Council on Medical Student Education in Pediatrics (COMSEP), of which she was the founding president from 1992 to 1993. This group has grown exponentially, remaining a critical force in medical student education, and she is proud of the collaboration, cooperation, and camaraderie that it fosters among clerkship directors. She was also able to take this one step further and created the organization called ACE (Alliance for Clinical Education) through the Association of American Medical Colleges (AAMC), which brought together leadership from each of the clerkship specialty organizations. This group has also grown tremendously, and although she has not been a part of the organization for nearly twenty-five years, she says, "Just to hear that it is alive and well and that it has a life of its own and is really, I think, an important contributing body to medical education is pretty cool." Throughout her seventeen-year tenure as pediatric clerkship director, she published extensively on her trials and successes, really illuminating the importance and legitimacy of medical education research and the building of an educator portfolio, an important academic track in institutions today.

With her expertise and commitment to education, Dr. Sahler became an asset and key contributor to the Division of Adolescent Medicine's competitive Leadership Education in Adolescent Health (LEAH) program, which the division held for fifteen years. She helped Dr. Richard Kreipe write the first grant in 1997, for which they were funded—a process she says really helped the program solidify its educational approach. She served as the program's medicine clinical coordinator and evaluation coordinator and developed a sophisticated evaluation system that the grant reviewing body described as one of the best evaluation processes they had seen. Just as she had done with the clerkship, she knew the importance of testing and measuring results to see how well processes worked, and this system relied heavily on feedback from the trainees in order to make modifications as needed. She referred to it as a continuous QI system and laughed as she said, "I think we thought of 360-degree evaluations before 360-degree evaluations got a name." She is proud of the legacy of their LEAH graduates, many of whom have had robust careers in academia and have been instrumental in developing new or making important contributions and changes to existing programs.

Dr. Sahler has seen many changes occur in the field of adolescent medicine over the years, but a constant she has found is the advocacy and respect adolescent medicine providers have for their patients as they help them navigate the transition into and out of adolescence, which she believes can be felt by the adolescents and is an important part of their growing up. She has been on the receiving end of many significant life moments her patients have chosen to share, oftentimes being the first person they have told. She brings a unique perspective with her background in palliative care, finding parallels in how she approaches conversations with the two groups: "One of the things I try to do is get people to put things into words so that they can realize that whatever the trauma is, whatever it is that they are going through, if they can speak it, it is out there, and it's just a word. And the word isn't going to hurt you. To say it, reveal it, and to find out people around you can be very supportive is really important."

This also applies to the conflict resolution counseling she does with families, noting adolescent medicine providers' important role in helping families work out the differences and problems that they are facing. She also finds that an important part of the Rochester program's success is the great deal of respect shared among its team members and their colleagues across the institution. "We don't shy away from difficult situations and our door is just about as open as it could be for everything," she said.

Looking to the future, she believes the field will continue to expand and get stronger as more continues to be learned about what is known to be unique to adolescents. Using an example from her work in pediatric hematology-oncology, the cancer prognosis and cure rates have historically been much lower in individuals between the ages of fifteen and thirty-nine. Especially for those between fifteen and twenty-six, she says it is extremely difficult because on a physiologic basis, certain cancers respond better to the treatments given to younger patients, rather than older patients. There is an important transition from pediatrics to medicine, which did not always consider that there are grey areas and a need to be very cognizant of whether the treatment being offered should be more pediatric-based or adult-based. While this has been recognized in certain cancer diagnoses in recent years, Dr. Sahler believes important realizations are to come in other disease processes, as well. In addition to the physiologic changes, she notes there are also philosophical changes when transitioning from a more protected pediatric care to the more autonomous adult medical care that can occur, ready or not, at the magic age of eighteen. "I think that we need to extend our horizons a little bit more," she said. "The challenge is there to really broaden the age range that we have experience with and can help patients through."

Always the student, Dr. Sahler most recently has decided to pursue her Master's degree in Medical Humanities and Bioethics and looks forward to broadening the reach of her career by doing so. In pursuing an additional degree, she is modeling the concept that we are all learners throughout our lifetimes.

Dr. Sahler's accomplishments and successes are varied and extensive and she has left her legacy in many substantive areas of pediatrics. From the national organizations she founded to improve and inform pediatric and medical education, to the critical role she played in helping obtain and foster Rochester's LEAH program, and to the tireless advocacy and support she has provided to patients and families in and out of Rochester, the fields of pediatrics and adolescent medicine have been markedly improved in major ways. Hers is a legacy marked by an energetic and passionate approach to questions, the answers to which will improve the task at hand: patient care, education, and research. Her role in the Division of Adolescent Medicine's history is and continues to be major, spanning over five decades of dedication. It is a stronger institution, department, and division because of Dr. Sahler's indelible influence on thousands of trainees and colleagues, and on society, locally, nationally, and internationally.

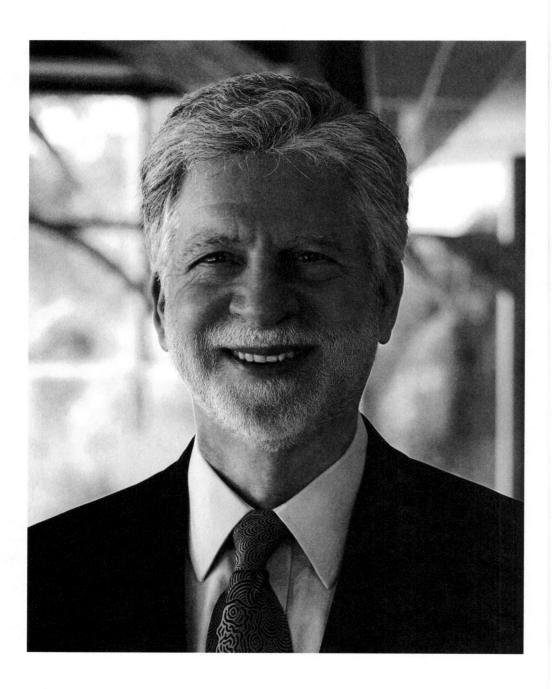

Chapter Twenty-Three

David M. Siegel, MD, MPH

As a quadruple board-certified physician in the specialties of pediatrics, internal medicine, pediatric rheumatology, and adolescent medicine, David Siegel has spent his influential career merging these interests and serving as a leader caring for adolescents and educating the next generation. A graduate of the University of Rochester's Internal Medicine and Pediatric residency programs and a General Academic Pediatrics fellowship program, he has spent almost the entirety of his inspiring career in Rochester. Prior to his retirement, he was the Northumberland Trust Professor of Pediatrics, the University of Rochester Pediatric Rheumatology Fellowship program director, and spent twenty years as the Edward H. Townsend Chief of Pediatrics at Rochester General Hospital/ Rochester Regional Health (RGH/RRH) (1999–2019).

Siegel was born in northern California where his family lived until he was ten years old before relocating to North Carolina. His father was a pediatrician who was committed to public health, activism, and social justice, leading him to pursue his Master of Public Health (MPH) at the University of California at Berkeley (while still practicing general pediatrics), where David and his siblings remember joining their parents at demonstrations and marches fighting for equality. It was 1964, the year of the Civil Rights Act, when his father accepted a job in the School of Public Health at the University of North Carolina (UNC) at Chapel Hill and the Siegel family moved to the South. Dr. Siegel remembers much turmoil, as it was the first year that the city's schools were not segregated. His family once again became involved with activism, but on a more tangible level—"It was a chance to take what in California had been meaningful, but more abstract, and really try to do something," he said. Siegel remained in Chapel Hill for college, and when it became time to apply for medical school, although he wanted to broaden his experiences, he said the high quality and in-state economics of UNC could not be surpassed. "So, I stayed, but I told myself, 'when I'm done with medical school, I've got to leave,'" he said with a laugh.

During medical school, Siegel became interested in interacting with people about their experiences, emotions, and mental health, causing him to consider pursuing psychiatry as a career. However, upon the advice of a friend and mentor who was a psychiatry resident at Duke University, he decided to pursue both internal medicine and pediatrics. At the time, UNC and the University of Rochester held the reputation for being among the nation's strongest combined Medicine-Pediatric residency programs. Knowing he wanted to branch out of Chapel Hill for the remainder of his training, he only applied to Rochester, telling himself that if he was not accepted into the highly competitive combined program, he would start as an internal medicine intern and then attempt to pursue each specialty to create his own combined experience, which is exactly what he did. Shortly after beginning his internal medicine residency at Rochester, he approached Dr. Robert Hoekelman, the then chair of the Department of Pediatrics, and asked if he could obtain experience in pediatrics with the goal of achieving board certification eligibility. Dr. Hoekelman was amenable to this plan and scheduled Dr. Siegel when there were gaps in the pediatric resident assignments. Dr. Siegel also continued his internal medicine training when not rotating on pediatrics. Between the two residencies, he ended up completing what amounted to twenty months of an intern's schedule, as opposed to the standard twelve—a period of his life he remembers being extremely tiring, but rewarding.

Still interested in the psychosocial aspects of medicine, something clicked when he rotated on the adolescent medicine unit. He has fond memories of learning from Dr. Elizabeth McAnarney; Dr. Richard Kreipe, who was a fellow at the time; and Dr. Christopher Hodgman, a consulting psychiatrist. He admired the way Dr. Hodgman interacted with families and was able to get both teenagers and their parent(s) to open up to him. With Dr. Hodgman agreeing to serve as his preceptor/supervisor, Dr. Siegel constructed a dedicated rotation on the adolescent consulting psychiatry service, which gave him even more exposure to adolescent medicine and solidified his interest. Another experience that had a significant and lasting impact on his career was during his first rotation in internal medicine, which occurred at Monroe

Community Hospital where his preceptor, Dr. John Baum, was an internationally prominent rheumatologist and became an influential mentor for Dr. Siegel and inspired his interest in rheumatology.

As the end of his residencies neared, Dr. Siegel found himself wanting to learn more about research and population health, while continuing to gain exposure in his clinical interests of adolescent medicine and rheumatology. He pursued a General Pediatric Academic fellowship at the University of Rochester, which afforded him the opportunity for all of that—continuing his primary care clinics in both Pediatrics and Internal Medicine at RGH, while also researching stress and its effect on triggering arthritis in children.

Due to a lack of job opportunities at the university, Dr. Siegel's first career postfellowship was practicing at a primary care office in Riverton, New York, where he was exceptionally busy, seeing nearly forty pediatric and adult patients each day while also taking in-house calls at Genesee Hospital. Just as he was beginning to explore other opportunities, the chief of Pediatrics at RGH/RRH, Dr. Charles "Dav" Cook, contacted him. Dr. Kreipe would soon be moving back to the University, and given Dr. Siegel's experience and interest in taking care of adolescents, Dr. Cook asked him to come take over the adolescent program Dr. Kreipe had started at RGH/RRH.

In addition to leading the adolescent program, covering the inpatient service and the newborn nursery, precepting the ambulatory clinic, working in the emergency room, and traveling to the URMC each week for rheumatology duties, Dr. Siegel was also assigned to work as the pediatrician at the Mary M. Gooley Hemophilia Center for Western New York located at RGH/RRH. This role would end up providing some of the most significant moments of his career and inspire much of his future work, as the time he took over was right as human immunodeficiency virus (HIV) first emerged. Because of the numerous blood product (Factor VIII) transfusions that patients who had hemophilia received (each bleeding episode exposing the patient to tens of thousands of unique blood donors), nearly all patients tragically were infected with HIV and contracting AIDS. "This was a very difficult time," Dr. Siegel said. "It was a horrible tragedy that all these people were infected. And one of the things that was just so painful and distressing about it was that the treatment that we recommended (transfusions of Factor VIII as early as possible when there was any concern for bleeding) is what infected them." Dr. Siegel was determined to help make a difference. "We're in the thick of this and I'm thinking, 'Blood transfusions are giving people HIV, sex is giving people HIV, adolescents are exploring sex,'" he said. "I thought, 'I have to do something about this. We can't be in the middle of this terrible community health crisis and not try to be part of the solution.'" Thus, he began to think about how he could go into schools, talk to adolescents about HIV, and carry out research to develop the most effective intervention for influencing the sexual decision making of adolescents.

Working with health educators, school nurses, principals, and superintendents, while overcoming a good amount of pushback and controversy from the community, he was able to construct an innovative educational framework incorporating middle and high school students as peer educators, initially supported by funding from Monroe County and New York State. In addition, eventually, with the help of nurse researcher and methodologist, Marilyn Aten, PhD, RN (who helped found Rochester's first adolescent maternity project), with whom Dr. McAnarney strategically partnered him, he secured a prestigious National Institute of Mental Health (NIMH) grant that allowed them to continue this work of taking preventive action in schools. They were able to design a successful curriculum, an intervention that they published and was ultimately implemented in additional areas outside of Rochester, as well as enroll thousands of adolescents to longitudinally follow up over three years. He credits Dr. Aten (and the dedicated health educators who committed themselves to the study, Rochester AIDS Prevention Project for Youth) with much of this success. He remains grateful to Dr. McAnarney for introducing two individuals who could not be more different, but were both committed to the idea that "If there's a health problem regarding adolescents, let's do something." Dr. Siegel fondly looks back at this immersive time in his career when adolescent medicine was central to both his clinical and academic work.

Over the years, Dr. Siegel's career continued to grow, including becoming chief of Pediatrics at RGH/RRH, division chief of Pediatric Rheumatology at the URMC Department of Pediatrics, and Rheumatology Fellowship program director. However, through each of his new commitments and responsibilities, he remained invested in adolescent health, continuing to work in the adolescent medicine clinic at RGH/RRH, through which all Rochester adolescent medicine fellows rotate. Due to his background in rheumatology, which led to many referrals for patients experiencing aches and pains, he was able to expose rotating medical students, residents, and adolescent medicine fellows to what he describes as a unique "musculoskeletal adolescent milieu." Further, when the American Board of Pediatrics declared adolescent medicine and rheumatology as board-certified specialties in 1991 and 1992, respectively, he pursued the alternative pathway they put forth, which allowed him to provide historical proof of his work in each area and to sit for each board examination. He ultimately received official board certification in both subspecialties.

Reflecting on the field of adolescent medicine, Dr. Siegel remarks on the important need it filled by closing the gap that existed in adolescent care, as neither pediatricians nor internists were particularly passionate about caring for this population. The group of pioneers who made adolescent medicine possible included Rochester's Dr. McAnarney. "The field made a difference because it became a healthcare home for these young people's needs, as well as a place to generate knowledge," he said. "I think it will remain a central pillar of pediatrics as a subspecialty and training. This is a core principle in taking care of kids."

As he looks back on his career, Dr. Siegel says he feels extremely grateful. "If I can spend my time in work doing something that is meaningful to me and makes me feel that I am contributing to something important, then that's pretty lucky," he said, noting that oftentimes people work to make a living, but derive deeper meaning from the "other stuff." "Everybody has different things that gratify them; but for me, I felt like, 'Wow, I get to go to work every day and do something that for me really matters.'"

Dr. Siegel has made profound contributions to adolescent health in Rochester and beyond through his varied clinical, academic, and teaching activities, while offering important and unique insight through his multispecialty background. A physician and academician with diverse training and areas of scholarly interest, he has played an important role in Rochester's adolescent program and continues to inspire the next generation. Dr. Siegel is a remarkable leader in several domains: adolescent medicine, pediatric rheumatology, and nurturing and assuring that the next generation of trainees participate in serious academic activities, while remaining true to one's goals and aspirations. His colleagues, patients, and families have benefited greatly from his wisdom and talents.

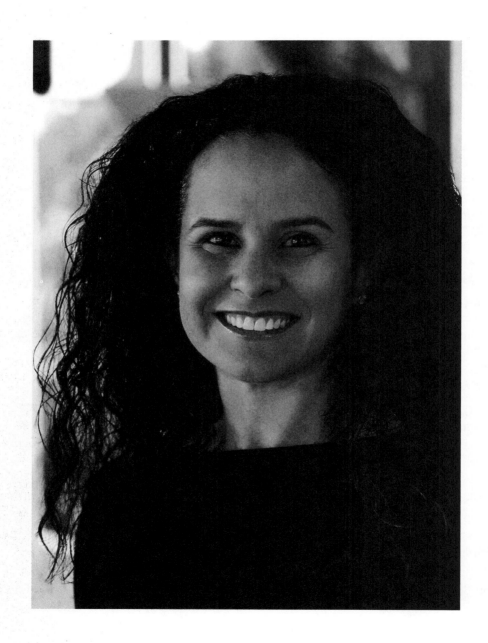

Chapter Twenty-Four

TAYLOR B. STARR, DO, MPH

Taylor Starr did not always know she wanted to be an adolescent medicine physician, but as soon as she learned the field existed, there was nothing else she could imagine doing. Growing up, she hoped she would find a career that she truly loved—and that is what she has done. As a talented clinician, committed educator, and inspiring mentor, Dr. Starr is an associate professor of Pediatrics and has been a valued member of Rochester's Adolescent Medicine Division since 2009.

Growing up in Queens, which she jokingly refers to as "the real New York," Starr spent much of her youth as a competitive gymnast. When she was in eighth grade, her science class piqued her interest in medicine. Her father, who was in real estate before the market crash, had recently become a funeral director—something that mortified her adolescent self. It was now the closest experience to studying medicine that was accessible to her, so she began to shadow him at work. At her young age, she thought orthopedic surgeons were the physicians who took care of athletes, and so, as an athlete herself, Starr aspired to do that. She headed to the University of Rochester for her undergraduate education and while there, she worked at University Health Service (UHS) as a peer health educator. She thoroughly enjoyed discussing health topics with her peers and was inspired to pursue a Master of Public Health (MPH) degree, for which she returned to New York City and attended Columbia University.

While in graduate school, she had a part-time job at the front desk of a large Obstetrics-Gynecology practice through the Albert Einstein College of Medicine. She received many phone calls from parents inquiring whether the providers at the practice cared for teenagers. While caring for patients of this age group, she learned it was not a main focus of the physicians and mid-wives. Dr. Starr thus identified a need for adolescent health care and hoped to one day become an obstetrician-gynecologist caring exclusively for teens. With this newfound passion, she set her sights again on medical school. Her former coach, who was a great mentor, had received his medical degree as an osteopath. Starr believed that her ideals aligned with the philosophy of osteopathic medicine—treating the person as a whole—and attended Lake Erie College of Osteopathic Medicine in Erie, Pennsylvania.

Her goal remained the same in medical school—to become an obstetrician-gynecologist for teens, less focused on obstetrics and more on sexual and reproductive health. While on a shift in the emergency room, she asked her attending preceptor if she could see any teenagers. Intrigued, the attending asked her about her interests, and she told him her plan. He looked at her and said, "Actually what I think you want to do is adolescent medicine." This was the first time she had heard of the field. Her preceptor said that she should speak with Dr. Warren Seigel, a well-known adolescent medicine physician, and they called him on the telephone together. "The second I got on the phone with him, something clicked," she said. "Anytime an adolescent medicine person talks to another adolescent medicine person, they click—it's like you're with your people." She had never felt this way before and after speaking with Dr. Seigel, she promptly set up an elective with him at Coney Island Hospital and began learning how to pursue an adolescent medicine fellowship.

Taylor decided to become a pediatrician, but she laughs, remembering how her resumé was completely devoid of pediatric interests. "I felt like I needed to lie my way into pediatric residency," she said. However, during her interviews, as she expressed her desire to care for adolescents, she felt welcomed immediately and realized programs were pursuing such candidates, as not every pediatrician wanted to take care of this unique age group. She ultimately attended Stony Brook University Hospital for residency from 2005 to 2009, where she worked with Dr. Joe Puccio, an adolescent medicine physician who trained with Dr. Seigel. Dr. Starr thrived and felt that powerful sense that she had a purpose and direction, one for which she could not wait. She also realized her passion for teaching others and went on to become a chief resident.

During one of her rotations, a fellow encouraged her to look at Leadership Education in Adolescent Health (LEAH) programs for fellowship, so she applied to LEAH programs throughout the country, including the University of Rochester. She visited other institutions first and came very close to signing with a program in the Midwest. However, when she visited Rochester, it immediately felt like a great fit. She remembers that Dr. Richard Kreipe, the division chief at the time, followed up Dr. Starr's interview visit with "amazing emails that were validating" and that made her feel like he truly listened to her. The location was also ideal, as she and her husband had just welcomed their son six weeks prior to her interview and Rochester would not be too far away from family. As Dr. Starr finished her fellowship, it was always her intent to return to Stony Brook to work with Dr. Puccio, which the Pediatrics chair even promised aloud during her residency graduation. Little did she know the hold Rochester would have on her and the career on which she was about to embark.

Dr. Starr took advantage of the diverse opportunities offered to her in fellowship, gaining experience and falling in love with all aspects of adolescent medicine, especially caring for patients who have eating disorders. While it was not something she originally thought that she would be doing, she said the training she received in caring for these patients was so exemplary that a new passion was born. There is an historical strength in the eating disorder program in Rochester, and Dr. Starr says that while the training is certainly diverse, that fact has not changed. "You do not leave here without being an expert," she said. In fact, the clinical work she does to help patients and families recover from eating disorders continues to be what she is most proud of accomplishing in her career.

The fellowship program also fostered her interest in educating patients, families, peers, and trainees, affording her the ability to take graduate courses at the university's school of education. "A very rich part of our institution is how diverse the expertise is across campuses," she said. "When we look and go out of our silos, we can really do neat cross-disciplinary work." Her scholarly work focused on educating providers, and she believes her main growth in fellowship was finding that niche for herself, which has remained a passion. In fact, in 2017, she became an associate medical director of the world's first and only Project ECHO (Extension for Community Healthcare Outcomes) program dedicated to eating disorders, which meets monthly with providers across New York State and beyond to provide education. It is a multidisciplinary group, including physicians, nurses, social workers, registered dieticians, and mental health providers.

As her fellowship graduation approached in 2012, it became clear to Dr. Starr and her family (who were now a family of four after welcoming their daughter during fellowship) just how special their time in Rochester was, and they had second thoughts about leaving. Aside from the extremely difficult task of telling their families they would not be returning home, she said accepting a faculty position in Rochester "was a no-brainer on every level—on my career, on the workplace, on outside the workplace, on family, on marriage, on fun, on mental and physical well-being."

As a junior attending, Dr. Starr wrestled with the overwhelming task of narrowing her focus, something she said she could not have done without the remarkable mentorship she received—both in fellowship and as a faculty member. "Pediatrics here at the University of Rochester sends a message of how important and valued mentorship is. It's engrained that you have mentors for all different parts of your life, and they're all equally important and can change over time." She said having that permission to shift course helped her immensely, as she realized she would change as a person, as an educator, and as a physician, and it is a sentiment that now guides her role as mentor to residents and fellows. In her early attending years, her mentors really helped her identify which opportunities benefited her career goals and helped her define her niche—eating disorders and education.

She acknowledges how these early opportunities and relationships she fostered allowed her to reach certain leadership levels—from medical director of an inpatient unit, 8 South, and the Eating Disorder Program at the Golisano Children's Hospital, to most recently an associate program director (APD) for Rochester's Pediatric and Medicine-Pediatrics Residency programs. This was a role she had been interested in for some time, so when a position opened up, and with encouragement from her division chief and mentors, she applied. As she interviewed for the APD position, she felt similarly as to when she was interviewing for residency—did she really fit? After all, she had never perceived herself professionally as a classical pediatrician. The program welcomed that diversity, however, and appreciated that Dr. Starr had an important role. Adolescent medicine provides a strong background for working with medical trainees. As the only subspecialist APD, she reaches trainees who have broad, creative career aspirations, much like herself in residency. It is a role that has brought her great joy and pride.

Throughout her career, Dr. Starr has witnessed great growth in the field of adolescent medicine and in Rochester's program. Since her fellowship, the division's gender health services have grown, reaching nearly the same percentage of patients as the division's longstanding eating disorders program. She believes it has become a real strength of the division, in which every provider is involved in delivering this important care. She has also seen improvement on a national level in meeting the sexual and reproductive health care needs of adolescents regarding long-acting reversible contraception (LARC), as well as in the transition of care of young people from pediatric care to adult care. Dr. Starr is extremely proud of the work their group has accomplished with medical and nursing colleagues in adult medicine to create a program that meets the needs of adult patients who require medical hospitalization secondary to complications from eating disorders. There is now a protocol and formal collaboration with medical and nursing colleagues in adult medicine, something new to the institution and one of a kind in the country. She is proud of the teamwork that occurred to close this gap.

Teamwork is quintessential to the program. "When I think of Rochester Adolescent Medicine, I think of a dynamic family of providers who have various passions and a commitment to the health and well-being of all adolescents in this world. I think of a team of the most supportive colleagues of whom one could dream," she said. Looking to the future, Dr. Starr views adolescent medicine as the guiding force in ensuring adolescents receive equitable and accessible healthcare. "I think we are the providers who make sure of that."

Although Dr. Starr humbly says she still feels junior, she has made great strides in the field of adolescent medicine and is now inspiring and educating the next generation of physicians and other health care providers. She has experienced many successes thus far in her career, including reaching that important goal she set as an adolescent herself—to find a career that she truly loves. Dr. Starr has grown into one of the outstanding role models and mentors to the next generation of trainees and adolescents. Her many skills are being applied toward clinical care, teaching, and administration of training programs for all levels of trainees and throughout the Eating Disorder program.

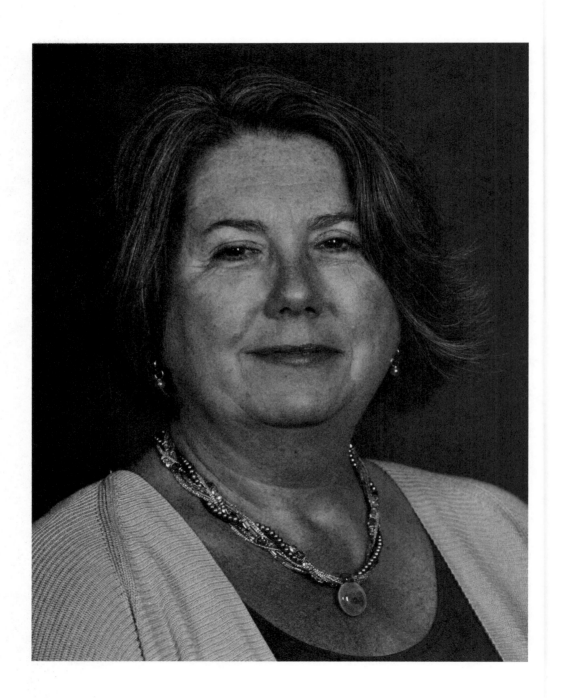

Chapter Twenty-Five

Helene Thompson-Scott, CNM, MS

The multidisciplinary nature of Rochester Adolescent Medicine is an important component to its rich history and success, and is evident by examining the career of midwife Helene Thompson-Scott and her influence on the program. She has held a critical role within the Rochester Adolescent Maternity Program (RAMP) for over thirty years, greatly affecting the lives of countless adolescents and their families.

Thompson-Scott is a Rochester native and graduate of Gates Chili High School where her interest in science developed. She attended Wheaton College for her undergraduate education. She decided to pursue nursing and attended nursing school at a small program outside of Chicago, West Suburban Hospital School of Nursing, and later received a Bachelor of Science in Nursing (BSN) from Rush University in Chicago. However, while returning to Rochester during her summer breaks, she worked at a summer camp for emotionally disturbed children, which had a profound impact on the trajectory of her career. "I was like a jack-of-all trades," she said with a laugh, noting that she had a bus license that allowed her to pick up the children in their neighborhood, but also had a natural ability to work with adolescents. The camp director realized this and assigned her to the adolescent girls' group. Upon her graduation from nursing school, she was unaware of positions that would allow her to work with the adolescent age-group in which she was most interested, so she followed another passion of hers and began her career in obstetrics, where she worked for ten years before she and her husband decided to move back to Rochester.

When she returned to Rochester, she learned of RAMP, which was run through the University of Rochester's Division of Adolescent Medicine, and thought, "This is right up my alley," given her obstetrics background and passion for working with adolescents. She ended up securing a job as an obstetrics nurse at Strong Memorial Hospital (SMH), but when she learned that RAMP was hiring a nurse, she said she literally ran from her unit on the second floor up to the fourth floor where the Department of Pediatrics was located. She remembers rushing into the office asking, "Is it too late?" It turned out they had finished their interviews, but after Thompson-Scott explained her interest and background, they brought her in to talk to someone. Later that afternoon, she received a call asking her to come for a formal interview the next day, and the rest is history. She served as a nurse in the program for nine years before ultimately becoming a midwife and joining the University Midwifery Group. She remained committed to RAMP, delivering the babies of teenage mothers and serving as director of the program.

While working as a nurse with RAMP, she developed strong relationships with her patients, so much so that they often wanted her to be present when they delivered their babies. This inspired her to develop her career even more and become a midwife, a role she has held since 1996. She attended Rochester's program for her Master of Science (MS) in Midwifery and completed her internship in Tucson, Arizona, with the Yaqui Indian Tribe, a unique experience she describes as a combined clinical and anthropological study. As a midwife, she is able to provide a full range of gynecological and obstetrical care with the exception of surgery/cesarean sections. The Midwifery Group at the University of Rochester sees approximately 500 deliveries each year for a diverse population, including adolescents—thus, each midwife in the practice is comfortable taking care of this age group and now shares in the RAMP director role to get to know the families ahead of delivery.

Throughout Thompson-Scott's time working with RAMP and Adolescent Medicine, she participated in several initiatives and programs that greatly affected the lives of young adolescent parents and their babies. One such program was called "Young Families," which involved going on home visits alongside a social worker, longitudinally following the mothers and babies over a period of two years. In addition to medical care, they also provided food, transportation, and any other needs the families had. It was also a time to help introduce and support breastfeeding, which at the time was a bit controversial with the teenage population. In fact, she believes one of her greatest contributions was the education she provided around breastfeeding, to both the adolescent mothers and their family support systems, which ultimately increased the rate. "There weren't yet lactation specialists in [the Department of] Obstetrics-Gynecology at that point, so we increased our breastfeeding rates with just education, giving people permission to breastfeed their babies, and then helping them if they needed help," she said. Through the Young Families program, they also saw success decreasing the teen pregnancy rate, which she attributes to being able to reduce the recurrence rate. "It was a lot of work," she said—work that consisted of education, continuous contact and support with families, and even bringing Depo doses straight to the home if a patient missed an appointment and wanted to prevent pregnancy so she could remain in school and graduate.

Additionally, she developed courses that not only covered breastfeeding, but the entire childbirth process. "I designed classes, and they were great fun," she said, "I taught them anything that anybody would learn in a childbirth class. I didn't leave it out because they were adolescents." She found working with adolescents was always fun, stemming all the way back to her summer camp experience. "Adolescents are learning and changing, but that doesn't mean it can't be fun and silly and goofy," she said. She employed this mentality when planning her birthing classes, recounting memories of making models of cervixes out of Play-Doh (and making the Play-Doh from scratch, a recipe the adolescents could then share with their children someday).

Helene was also part of a group of RAMP providers, including nurse practitioners Suzanne Fullar and Mary Sprick, who developed a program called "Group Prenatal Care." This program brought together pregnant adolescents who had similar due dates and provided education, including teaching them how to listen to the baby's heartbeat with a special stethoscope, take each other's weight and blood pressure, and then log the information. "They kept their own charts and also took care of each other," she said, noting that it helped create a bond and friendship among them. They would then formally gather again as a group after their babies were born, and many continued their relationship and support of each other beyond the class. This framework ended up being used in the development of a large, national group-based prenatal program called "Centering Pregnancy," which an individual outside of Rochester patented after further developing and expanding the concept, but always included the Rochester program in her references. Helene still participates in prenatal care, and while the COVID-19 pandemic put a hold on in-person gatherings, she hopes to one day create an additional group centered on menopause, a concept inspired by the mothers of her patients. Many of her adolescent participants would bring their mothers to the class, who would have questions about their own health. "They are in a group setting and everyone is freely talking, and I end up starting to see them as patients," she said. "They told me, 'I want a group for me,' which is a really good idea!"

Ms. Thompson-Scott has witnessed the impact that Adolescent Medicine and its programming has had on the community and the overall health of teenagers. "I'm proud that we were able to have good outcomes for our patients—we had healthy babies and healthy moms," she said. Additionally, this programming not only helped adolescents through their pregnancies, but also improved their health afterwards. "These teenagers were pregnant for a very short time of their life, but they were still adolescents and still needed healthcare," she said, explaining that the sexually transmitted infections (STIs), contraception, and pregnancy services that Adolescent Medicine provided served as a gateway for getting care. She was also involved with community programs, including school-based health centers, the Center for Youth, and teen community center, Threshold, where she ran prenatal programs and saw any pregnant patient that pursued care through the clinic. "Adolescent Medicine really infiltrated the community at every level," she said. "Wherever there were adolescents, the Division of Adolescent Medicine had people!"

When she thinks of Rochester Adolescent Medicine, she said she thinks of a community presence and a group of problem solvers, noting that she and her colleagues ask themselves "How can we come together and solve this problem? What can we create to make it work or make something different happen?" She also marvels at the amount of expertise that is readily available.

"An adolescent could be pregnant, but she has an eating disorder; or an adolescent could be pregnant, but she has a gastrointestinal disease," she said. "We had so many experts at our fingertips because they were so present." Although she no longer works under the umbrella of Adolescent Medicine (as the teenage pregnancy rate in Rochester decreased, RAMP shifted to the Department of Obstetrics-Gynecology, as there wasn't as great a need in Adolescent Medicine), she still relies on that expertise and stays in touch with the adolescent medicine providers with whom she worked so closely for years. "It is really special to be able to count on those previous relationships in order to coordinate care for patients," she said.

Helene certainly found her calling, as she has been able to spend her career overlapping her two worlds of obstetrics and working with adolescents, and has made a profound impact in doing so. The University's Obstetrics and Gynecology, Adolescent Medicine groups, and greater Rochester community, have surely benefited from her ingenuity, leadership, and passion.

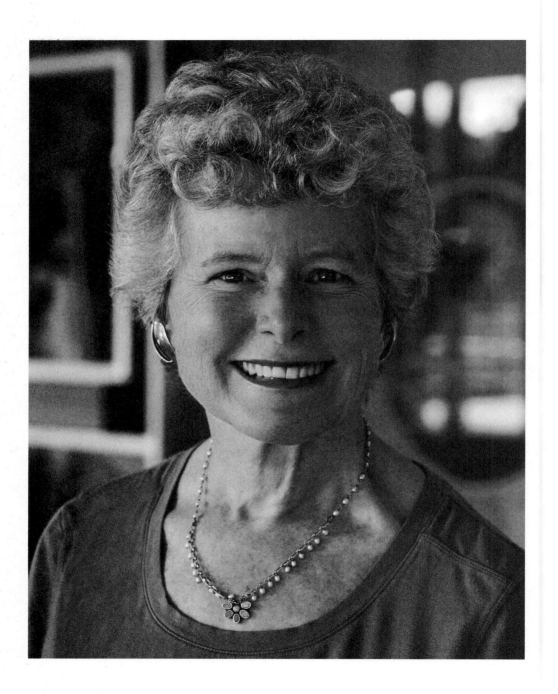

Chapter Twenty-Six

JANE I. TUTTLE, PhD, RN, FNP-BC, FAANP

Jane Tuttle has devoted her career to improving the health of adolescents and families, and inspiring the next generation to do so as well. As a professor emerita of Clinical Nursing and Pediatrics, she has served as a leader within the University of Rochester School of Nursing and Department of Pediatrics, where she has been an integral part of the Rochester Adolescent Medicine team. Her leadership and contributions to the division's Leadership Education in Adolescent Health (LEAH) program and Teen-Tot clinic have been a critical part of each program's success. Even after her official retirement in 2017, she has remained involved with teaching and mentoring at the School of Nursing, advocating for adolescent health, particularly transitions to adult care, and helping ignite a passion in others for working with adolescents.

Tuttle was born and raised in Rochester, New York, and it was her love for science and working with people that led her to pursue a career in nursing. She attended Monroe Community College for her Associate of Applied Science (AAS) degree in Nursing in 1974 followed by State University of New York (SUNY) Buffalo for her certificate as a Pediatric Nurse Associate/Practitioner. "I loved to learn and went on from there," she said. She received her Bachelor of Science in Nursing (BSN) from the University of Rochester in 1979, which is when she was first introduced to the Department of Pediatrics and the Division of Adolescent Medicine. She said she gravitated toward adolescent health, pursuing both clinical and scholarly opportunities within the hospital and community, including a multiyear project with the Rochester

City School District. Following her graduation, she spent a few years practicing in Washington, DC, before returning to the University of Rochester to pursue her masters in primary care nursing (FNP).

As part of her master's program, Tuttle took a course in adolescence taught by Adolescent Medicine nurse, the late Marilyn Aten, PhD, RN, who would become an important mentor to Tuttle. During this time, she also completed a rotation in the adolescent clinic with Dr. Richard Kreipe where her passion for working with adolescents continued to grow. She has fond memories of monthly meetings at the Princess Restaurant with Kreipe and all of the adolescent providers in the community to discuss adolescent health, including current challenges, triumphs, and the recent literature. She also understood the importance of the field on a personal level, as she was raising her son, who was an adolescent at the time. "I knew how important it was. Teenagers are definitely underserved and misunderstood," she said, acknowledging how thankful she was for a group of providers doing their best to meet the needs of this population and help them thrive.

Upon receiving her master's degree, she and her son moved to New Haven, Connecticut, after she obtained a faculty position at Yale University School of Nursing, with a part-time nurse practitioner position at Guilford Pediatrics. Interested in furthering her education, she began a PhD program in family studies at the University of Connecticut. Her dissertation, "Family Support, Adolescent Individuation, and Substance Abuse," surveyed over 1,900 adolescents and examined how they navigated individuation and development of autonomy within the family and how that impacted their choices around drug and alcohol use. "It was a great experience, and from there, everything I have done has been about teenagers," she said. Upon receiving her doctorate, and longing to return to a more research-intensive environment, she ran into the late Dr. Marilyn Aten at a Society for Adolescent Health and Medicine (SAHM) meeting—"And the next thing you know, I'm back in Rochester," she said with a smile.

The Division of Adolescent Medicine was applying for the Maternal and Child Health Bureau (MCHB)-funded LEAH program and Dr. Tuttle was asked to serve as the nursing discipline coordinator, which is a role she held for the fifteen years that the program was funded. In this capacity, she led and served as the primary advisor to the cohort of nursing trainees. LEAH was comprised of five core disciplines—medicine, nursing, nutrition, psychology, and social work—that worked collaboratively through didactic, clinical, and community leadership activities. "LEAH was such a great program. The inter-professional approach looked at the whole picture—not just the health, but social, economic, and political influences on youth. It was really rich," she said. "It was fifteen years of wonderful training for folks, and we have many graduates who are making a big impact." Her nursing graduates have earned accolades for their work, which includes conducting international research on human immunodeficiency virus (HIV) and serving in leadership roles, such as assistant dean of Diversity and Inclusion for the School of Nursing. Tuttle later served as the nursing discipline coordinator for the department's Leadership Education in Neurodevelopmental Disabilities (LEND) program for seventeen years, where her primary focus was the transition to adult healthcare for youth with special healthcare needs. She advocated on a national level to embed such training in medical and nursing curricula, which has begun to occur, including within the University of Rochester's Developmental and Behavioral Pediatrics program.

In addition to the LEAH program, Jane was extremely involved with the Division's Teen-Tot Clinic, which provided simultaneous care for adolescent mothers and their babies. She helped lead the program for over twenty years with an Adolescent Medicine faculty partner, Dr. Cheryl Kodjo, and it remains among her proudest contributions. The program worked in close conjunction with the Rochester Adolescent Maternity Program (RAMP), which Jane describes as "phenomenal." In fact, she has earlier ties to its work, as she analyzed data from RAMP for her master's thesis, "A Study of Factors Associated with Effective Contraceptive Behavior in Adolescent Women." She had the opportunity to witness similar adolescent maternity programs elsewhere in the country and finds something special about Rochester's. She quotes the University's motto, *Meliora,* meaning "ever better," while also attributing the University's history with the development of the biopsychosocial model. "Rochester Adolescent Medicine is a shining example of using the biopsychosocial model to address health challenges," she said. "I think we exemplify that when we think of working with adolescents. Anything that has to do with adolescent health really has that model at its heart." Something else she has found unique to Rochester is the emphasis and value placed on multidisciplinary care. She is grateful to Drs. Marilyn Aten and Elizabeth McAnarney for helping her obtain a secondary appointment in the Department of Pediatrics. "People who are not physicians get to be a part of the pediatric faculty, and the fact that we're valued and embraced in real ways means a lot," she said. "That's another thing that's remarkable about Rochester."

Dr. Tuttle has also served as a leader within the University of Rochester School of Nursing, where she was the director of the Family Nurse Practitioner (FNP) program for nearly twenty years. Since retirement, she has remained involved, particularly through teaching and advising. She enjoys training others and endorsing the field of adolescent health. "I'm always promoting people not being afraid to work with adolescents—helping them overcome barriers and feel more comfortable and able to engage effectively with teenagers and their families in the larger context," she said. While she has certainly made an impact on the health of adolescents and their families at the clinical level, she is also proud of training others to do so as well. Her research contributions have also made an impact in the field. She published the results of both her master's thesis and PhD dissertation, as well as several other articles about adolescent health, and led a research team funded by the National Institutes of Health (NIH) to study group interventions for at-risk adolescents (Teen Club and Positive Adolescent Life Skills).

Dr. Tuttle has watched the field grow and change throughout her more than forty years of practice, including what she refers to as "movement from problem-oriented to strength-based care of adolescents and consideration of their larger context of family, friends, school, and society—especially the explosion of social media," she said. "It is definitely recognized that family is critical to the adolescent's development and well-being." She recognizes the effects that a global pandemic and divisive political climate have had on modernday adolescents, especially related to mental health, but remains optimistic about the future. "Youth are our future and that is increasingly recognized," she said. "I'd like to think we'll continue to fund for adolescent health training and for programs that benefit kids and help them be their best selves and to grow through these adverse things."

Dr. Tuttle has accomplished much throughout her career and has made a profound impact on the health of adolescents and their families, as well as on the education of future adolescent healthcare leaders. Her commitment to adolescent health and the programs and services offered in Rochester has resulted in a lasting legacy for countless patients, families, and trainees.

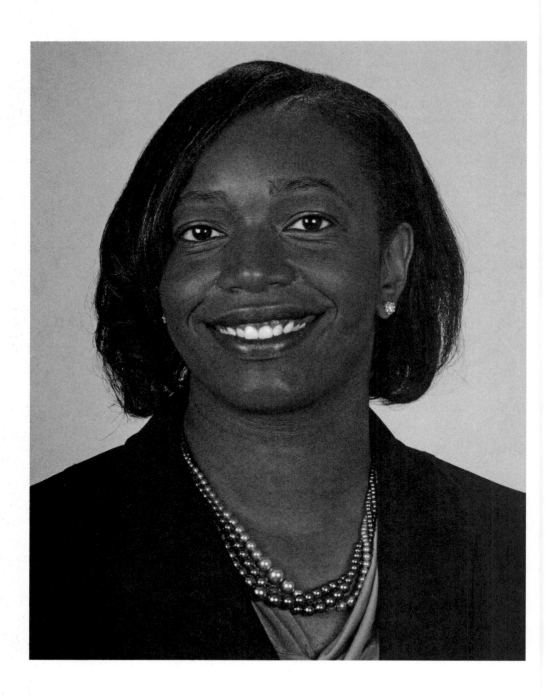

Chapter Twenty-Seven

LeKeyah N. Wilson, MD

LeKeyah Wilson is a proud alumna of the University of Rochester, three times over, as a graduate of the University of Rochester School of Medicine and Dentistry (2007), Pediatrics Residency program (2010), and Adolescent Medicine Fellowship program (2013). She has spent her entire career caring for adolescents, specifically invested in their mental and behavioral health, and she has made profound contributions to the greater Rochester community.

Wilson is a second generation Rochesterian and a graduate of Penfield High School. She remembers first dreaming of becoming a pediatrician when she was in the fifth grade, and as she progressed through school was counseled to seek experience in hospitals. Thus, during high school, she volunteered as a candy striper at the University of Rochester Medical Center's (URMC) pediatric infusion clinic, which solidified her interest in medicine, and specifically pediatrics.

She attended Howard University in Washington, DC, where she took premedical courses and volunteered at Howard University Hospital. When applying to medical school, she planned to remain in Washington, DC. However, her parents begged her to consider coming back home. She applied to and was interviewed at the University of Rochester School of Medicine and Dentistry (URSMD), and much to her surprise and her parents' contentment, fell in love with the institution. "I didn't want to like it, but I ended up loving it," she said with a laugh. What struck LeKeyah on her interview day was the apparent camaraderie among the classmates. It was an exam day for the students, and yet they seemed calm and happy, she remembers. "It was a peculiar vibe," she said. "Why aren't people cramming? Why aren't people worried? My thoughts were, 'Okay, if they are feeling like this before an exam, then the medical school must be doing something right that keeps the students really happy." She ended up staying for her pediatrics residency and adolescent medicine fellowship. The warmth and feeling of genuine camaraderie is a theme that was carried throughout all stages of her training.

It was during medical school when Wilson realized adolescent medicine could be a great fit for her. As she rotated through various disciplines, she found herself drawn to the behavioral health aspects of each, but she was not sure psychiatry was the right path for her. That is when she met Dr. Richard Kreipe, the division chief of Adolescent Medicine at the time, who suggested she pursue fellowship training. As she learned more from him, and met another Adolescent Medicine faculty member, Dr. Cheryl Kodjo (about whom she fondly remembers thinking, "I want to be like her when I grow up!"), her interest was piqued. She describes herself meeting these two adolescent medicine doctors and thinking, "Wow, they must be a part of an incredible division; I want to learn more about what they do."

She thought it was an incredible division during her time in medical school and residency, but learned to appreciate it even more when she was on the residency interview trail. As she discussed her budding interest in adolescent medicine with the various programs with which she interviewed, they would half-jokingly ask, "Why are you here? Rochester is known for Adolescent Medicine!" When it was time to apply for fellowship, she ultimately found Rochester's program to be the best fit. "The program was one that you can make your own and that's the piece that I really liked about it—being able to design your own electives and create your own focus," she said.

Dr. Wilson's primary interests during fellowship included mental health and youth violence. As she designed her research project focused on youth violence, she constructed a multidisciplinary scholarship oversight committee that included Dr. Michael Scharf, the division chief of Pediatric Psychiatry. She also completed electives in psychiatry, and became involved with the Rochester Youth Violence Partnership with Dr. Scharf and trauma surgeon, Dr. Mark Gestring. "The fellowship was so supportive of me going out and making those community connections," she said.

Another aspect of her fellowship experience that she remains very grateful for is the training she received through the Leadership Education in Adolescent Health (LEAH) grant, which the division held at the time. It gave her a breadth of experience in collaborating across disciplines, a skill she frequently calls upon in her career to this day. "I really think that time with LEAH has developed me into the type of physician that I am now," she said. "Something I truly took away from fellowship was communication skills, whether it was with adolescent patients, their families, other subspecialists, nursing care, or teams from behavioral health. Understanding where your families were coming from and understanding other perspectives—I think that is one of the arts of adolescent medicine."

Upon graduation from fellowship, Dr. Wilson joined adolescent medicine physician, Dr. David Siegel, at Rochester General Hospital/Rochester Regional Health (RGH/RRH), where he was then chief of Pediatrics. She describes it as a "hodge-podge" of a job with a combination of time spent on the pediatric inpatient unit and newborn nursery, ambulatory adolescent medicine clinic, and teaching activities. Additionally, during fellowship, Dr. Wilson completed an elective rotation with Dr. Stephen Webb, who oversaw multiple school-based health and youth detention centers in the city. Fortuitously, as she was lining up her postfellowship job at RGH, Dr. Webb was getting ready to retire and chose Dr. Wilson as his replacement. This ended up being the perfect complement to her job at RGH, the hospital through which these centers were run. In becoming the medical director for five school-based health centers (SBHCs) and two detention centers, Dr. Wilson served as the conduit that brought the hospital and centers closer together.

Something else Dr. Wilson brought to RGH/RRH, which she views as one of her greatest contributions, is that of NEXPLANON insertions. She led the initiative to train additional staff, who then would serve as preceptors to the pediatric residents and take this service to one of the SBHCs. "I truly believe in informed consent and having those options for our youth, versus just referring them elsewhere," she said. She is grateful for the opportunity she had in fellowship to receive training in this procedure, as she has been able to utilize that to make these notable advancements.

Dr. Wilson is still involved in each of her original inpatient, ambulatory, and teaching activities at RGH/RRH, although she has taken on more leadership roles, including her most recent promotion to medical director of Community Pediatrics and Wellness, something she credits to her fellowship training. "[Fellowship] allowed me to find my voice—my voice for myself and for my patients. And it has prepared me to be a leader," she said. "It's like they flipped a switch for us and said, 'You guys are natural-born leaders; let us give you the tools to help you navigate so that you can lead.'" Wilson said she has found herself speaking up more and having a seat at the table, something with which she was not always comfortable. "It really comes from experience and your training and a fellowship that believes in you. I felt very strongly that they believed in me. Whatever I wanted to do or accomplish, they would say, 'okay, how do we help you get there?'"

Dr. Wilson is most proud of her patient relationships, including the longevity of many. She recounts one such patient who followed her from fellowship to her practice at RGH/RRH, whom she treated through an early eating disorder, pregnancy, and afterwards. A few years later, she received a message from this patient thanking Dr. Wilson for believing in and encouraging her. The former patient detailed that she and her son are healthy and happy, crediting much of that to Dr. Wilson. "There's a part of me that feels like I don't deserve that credit, as they are the ones who do all the hard work," she said. "But it is a privilege to walk along with them as they go through that journey. I think of adolescence like that—it is a journey into adulthood. Sometimes you slip, sometimes you fall, and sometimes you elevate yourself. It is not just a trajectory straight up to being successful; it is more like a jagged line. And to watch adolescents hit that maturity level and be okay, I think that is awesome." It is these relationships and the impact they have on both patient and provider that has meant the most to her. "Your impact matters, your involvement matters, and you can truly make a difference from your bedside manner, the way you practice medicine, the way that you believe in your patients, and the way you encourage them," she said.

When reflecting on the field, Dr. Wilson believes that, with the increase in knowledge about adolescent medicine, adolescents are in turn receiving better care. When she sees a patient for the first time, she introduces herself and explains what she does. She says that oftentimes the parent or guardian will remark, "You deal with all of that? I needed one of you back when I was a teenager!" She feels that, by providing care on subject matters that may have not yet come to the surface, the adolescent medicine provider's role is important in normalizing and destigmatizing behaviors, especially those related to mental health. Further, through collaborations with the Department of Psychiatry and the TEACH program (psychiatric training for primary care providers), she says, "I think that definitely opened up everyone's eyes on providing behavioral health in primary care. I think adolescent medicine definitely helped pave that road." Reproductive healthcare is another area where she believes adolescent medicine has led the way—normalizing care in areas that were once considered taboo.

She says she has seen an increase in awareness of adolescent medicine at the hospital level, as well, especially when someone from the specialty is included in discussions of new guidelines, service lines, administration, and so on for pediatric care. A recent example is policies for the handling of electronic health records and issues of access. "We do a lot of advocacy," she said. "How do we protect [adolescents'] rights and make sure their rights are also being acknowledged? I think that's definitely something adolescent medicine has historically provided to the empowerment of youth."

Rochester Adolescent Medicine will always have a special place in Dr. Wilson's heart—"We'll always be family," she said, noting that she enjoys every chance to collaborate, including precepting the adolescent medicine fellows in her RGH adolescent clinic. She is proud of the legacy of the Rochester program, and remains in awe of the accomplishments and contributions that have come out of the division. "They are pioneers in their field," she said, noting the feeling of admiration when picking up a textbook or review article authored by one of her mentors. "You're like, 'I didn't know I was in the presence of a celebrity' because they are so humble about their accomplishments in life and they have achieved so much. It's just an honor to be trained by them." The open-door policy provided by everyone, including Dr. Elizabeth McAnarney, Department of Pediatrics Chair Emerita, and the life lessons and practical skills surrounding work-life balance that were provided by Dr. Shellie Yussman, Dr. Wilson's fellowship program director, remain key memories of her fellowship. "It was just a really great experience—so many lessons learned beyond the medicine," she said.

Dr. Wilson's leadership in the areas of adolescent mental health and youth violence, compassionate care creating lasting relationships with her patients, and commitment to advocating for and empowering adolescents is evident in each role she undertakes. Her hometown and her university are justly proud of Dr. Wilson's presence over time and training in the community. The ultimate gift is that Dr. Wilson returned to Rochester and is now leading the way for young people in medicine and in her community. She deserves the respect and admiration earned within her hometown and beyond.

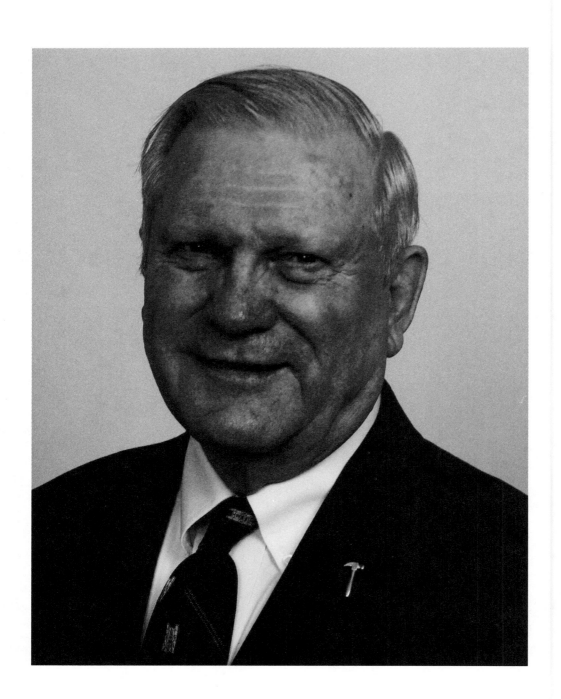

Chapter Twenty-Eight

W. SAM YANCY, MD

William Samuel "Sam" Yancy has a rich history within the field of adolescent medicine, contributing greatly to its history, recognition, and growth. Mentored by Dr. Stanford Friedman, the founding director of Rochester's Adolescent Medicine program, Dr. Yancy is a 1971 graduate of the Adolescent Medicine and Behavioral Pediatrics fellowship program at the University of Rochester. He spent his career focusing on two passions—his general pediatrics practice and leadership in adolescent medicine academics and policymaking. An international leader, his contributions have brought new discoveries, programs, and initiatives that helped propel the field forward.

Yancy was born in a small town outside of Oxford, Mississippi. His family moved after the start of World War II to Richland, Washington, for his father's job with the Atomic Energy Commission. He remembers his kindergarten teacher greeting the class each morning with warnings to be careful of foreign objects that may be dropped on U.S. soil, and collecting cans for "Save the War." His family moved several times because of his father's job, returning to Mississippi before ultimately going to Falls Church, Virginia. Yancy's interest in medicine was piqued at an early age, as the father of his best friend in Mississippi was the only doctor in their small town of 2,500 people. "I admired him and decided that's what I wanted to do," he said. He attended Duke University in Durham, North Carolina for his undergraduate and medical educations, followed by one year of pediatrics training before heading to Rochester as a second-year resident. Interested in ambulatory pediatrics, he was drawn to the Rochester program's strong national reputation in that area and spent a year of training there. It was during this time that he also received his first introduction to the field of adolescent medicine.

While in Rochester, he found role models within the adolescent medicine group, including Drs. Stanford Friedman, Elizabeth McAnarney, and Philip Nader. Dr. Yancy remembers weekly developmental sessions arranged by Dr. Friedman, which covered topics from birth through adolescence. The format included a didactic session on the development of a certain age group, followed by observation of a faculty member interviewing and developmentally testing that age group. "It was an amazing experience to have that quality of education on a regular basis over a period of time," he said. "To not just hear about development and behavior, but to see it week-to-week."

Following his year in Rochester, he returned to Duke for his final year of residency training, and then entered the service, where he was stationed at Camp Pendleton in Southern California at a naval teaching hospital. Because of his exposure to adolescent medicine in Rochester, Dr. Yancy was asked to start a clinic for adolescents there, which became one of the first military adolescent programs in the country. Given his interest and desire to learn more about the field, he returned to Rochester after his service to pursue fellowship training.

Dr. Yancy remembers a unique educational offering in Rochester, which was that of being supervised and then debriefed by faculty of three different disciplines—pediatricians, psychiatrists, and psychologists. The trainees audiotaped their interviews with adolescent patients and then reviewed the recordings with at least two faculty from the different disciplines. "It was a tremendous way to learn about interviewing adolescents," he said. He also reflects that during his fellowship training, school health was just beginning to become prominent in some institutions, and Dr. Friedman arranged for the fellows to partake in counseling experiences in the Monroe County high schools. Dr. Yancy was encouraged to open a substance abuse clinic for the high school, which was met with resistance by the principal who did not believe a substance abuse problem existed. To identify the need, Yancy conducted a survey across all of the county high schools, which ended up being one of the largest surveys focused on substance abuse and attitudes among high school students in the country at the time. It confirmed the suspected substance abuse problem, and Dr. Yancy organized a clinic. Through his scholarly and clinical work, he was able to bring to light new information about adolescent substance abuse among teenage students, with a particular emphasis on the behavioral and attitudinal components, such as how they viewed the legality or illegality of various drugs.

Following his fellowship, Dr. Yancy returned to Duke University, citing the climate as a chief reason—"I had spent most of my life below the Mason-Dixon Line and I was not used to the weather up there," he said with a laugh. He was recruited to Duke to start an Adolescent Medicine training program, but was also able to continue his passion for general pediatrics, which remained important to him—the best of both worlds. "One of the most satisfying things I've had throughout my practice is watching families, both parents and children, grow and develop over a period of time," he said. "Probably one of the biggest milestones in my practice was when some of my former patients started bringing their children to see me."

In addition to his general practice, Dr. Yancy founded Duke's adolescent training program in 1971 and continued to lead the program for nearly thirty years, placing a focus on training residents in the behavioral aspects of pediatrics and adolescent medicine. The Rochester program had instilled in him the importance of lifelong teaching. "Almost everywhere I've been, people talk about education as a lifelong process and that you want to be a lifelong learner. Rochester was no different; they certainly emphasized that. But they also emphasized lifelong teaching," he said. "If we're going to learn new things, whether it's through clinical practice or research, we also need to disseminate that new knowledge so that others can benefit from what we have learned. I think that's something that stuck with me throughout my career."

Dr. Yancy was also significantly involved with the Society for Adolescent Health and Medicine (SAHM), holding various leadership positions, including executive secretary-treasurer (1978–1983) and president (1985–1986). He credits much of his involvement in the society to his time in Rochester, which has a strong legacy of SAHM leadership and participation since the society's inception. Dr. Yancy remarks that in addition to multiple past presidents and recipients of the prestigious Outstanding Achievement Award (Drs. Friedman and McAnarney), multiple Rochester pediatric faculty (Drs. Gilbert

Forbes and Robert Haggerty) served as invited Gallagher Lecturers. This is an esteemed invited lectureship named after Dr. J. Roswell Gallagher, the first SAHM president, who is credited with establishing the first Adolescent Medicine program in the country. Committed to the academic and policy-making aspects of adolescent medicine throughout his career, Dr. Yancy played a key role in the process of developing an official board-recognized subspecialty of adolescent medicine, and also made an international impact in Puerto Rico during his time as president of SAHM. In partnership with Dr. Friedman, he also served as a cofounder and president of the Society for Developmental and Behavioral Pediatrics.

Additionally, as the first board certified adolescent medicine physician in the state of North Carolina, Dr. Yancy established the Committee on Adolescent Health through the American Academy of Pediatrics (AAP) North Carolina Pediatric Society, as well as a Child Advocacy Committee in the city of Durham. "I was able to do a lot of things I would not have been able to do had I not been given opportunities through my experience in Rochester to become a certified adolescent medicine physician, and therefore be attractive to Duke to support me in doing these things," he said. When reflecting on his career, he said, "I would say the thing I am most proud of is that I was able to maintain a general practice and help children and parents grow and develop, and at the same time be involved in the academic aspects of adolescent medicine. I was able to participate in all of the kinds of things, including research and teaching, that you would not ordinarily do as a general pediatrician." Through his national involvement in the field, Dr. Yancy stayed in close contact with his Rochester colleagues throughout the years. "That kind of relationship extending for fifty years is a very warm feeling to have," he said. "I couldn't tell you all of the accolades that have been bestowed on all those people. They are fantastic people, but they are very important people to me because of their friendship, their mentorship, their companionship, and their willingness to help over a long period of time."

Dr. Yancy is proud of the growth he has witnessed in the field of adolescent medicine, remembering spending much time at the beginning of his career explaining what adolescent medicine specialists were doing to a population that did not understand why adolescents needed a specific focus.

"[Adolescents] were kind of a lost group of individuals that didn't get much attention," he said. "So, we spent a lot of time explaining what adolescent medicine was, and came to be recognized as a field that could have an impact on the lives of individuals in that age group." He said while there is and always will be room for improvement, he has certainly witnessed advancements from the standpoint of school health, counseling, substance abuse, adolescent pregnancy, eating disorders, and more. "None of those things would have had much attention at all if it hadn't have been for adolescent medicine physicians bringing that attention and bringing new information about those problems to the medical community," he said.

Dr. Yancy officially retired in 2005, but he still uses his talents to serve others. Trading in his stethoscope for a hammer, he spends his time helping to build twenty houses a year with Durham Habitat for Humanity. His legacy in the field of adolescent medicine stretches far and wide—a leader whose commitment to adolescent health, the growth of the field, and lifelong teaching through the dissemination of knowledge have contributed to important advancements and the health and well-being of adolescents throughout the world.

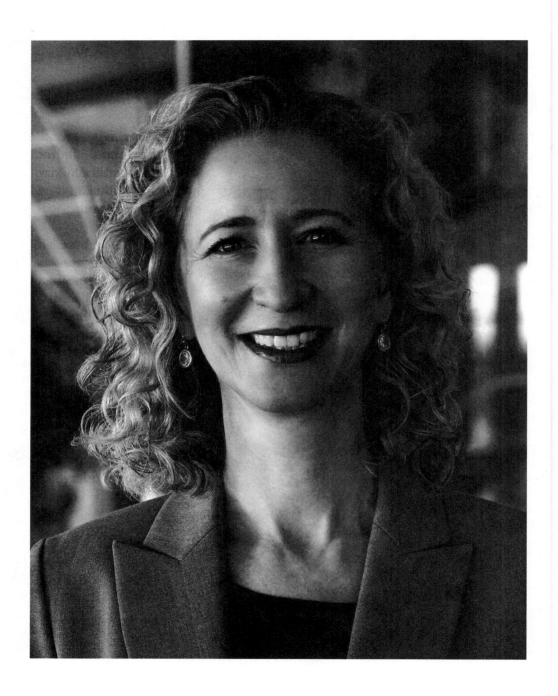

Chapter Twenty-Nine

Susan (Shellie) M. Yussman, MD, MPH

Susan (Shellie) Yussman, Professor of Pediatrics and Center for Community Health and Prevention, is a valued leader in the Division of Adolescent Medicine, currently serving as division chief and fellowship program director. Her early interests in advocacy and working with under-resourced youth are what led her to a career in adolescent medicine, and have remained a passion and focus of much of her professional work. She is a skillful mentor to fellows and faculty alike and has helped the Division of Adolescent Medicine grow, evolve, and expand its clinical services throughout the Western New York region.

Yussman grew up in Louisville, Kentucky. While many of her family members were businesspeople, teachers, attorneys, and doctors, they helped people in their various fields. Dr. Yussman recalls how her mother, a high school special education teacher, would step away from the dinner table to take telephone calls when her students needed assistance, and she remembers how students would thank her mother, their teacher, at graduations, for her mother's guidance. As early as middle school, she knew she wanted to help people by pursuing a career in medicine and live up to her mother's example. These childhood memories would become even more meaningful over the course of Dr. Yussman's career as she eventually taught residents and fellows, seeing them off at their own graduations.

Yussman attended Washington University in St. Louis, Missouri, for her undergraduate education, and while she took all of the premedical requirements, she had a love for literature and languages and was able to major in English literature and double minor in Spanish and biology. She continued to consider her career options throughout college, but ultimately decided to pursue the medical career of which she had always dreamed. "I was always interested particularly in young women's health and advocacy, and I felt like that would be a way that I could really make a difference," she said.

She returned to Kentucky for her medical education and attended the University of Louisville School of Medicine. She remarks that she encountered some challenging social dynamics, as she found her primary interests were not so common among medical students. However, she was able to find her niche when a mentor suggested adolescent medicine. Because her medical school did not have a strong adolescent medicine program in place at the time, she completed an elective rotation at the Medical College of Virginia at Virginia Commonwealth University with Dr. Richard Brookman, a well-respected national figure in adolescent medicine. She had found her calling.

Dr. Yussman pursued a pediatric residency and matched at Oregon Health and Science University (OHSU) where she had a wonderful experience. While there, she enjoyed working with under-resourced patients and families and she considers an off-campus elective working with the Indian Health Service on a Navajo reservation to be her favorite experience. She loved this work so much that she considered continuing her career with the Indian Health Service. However, she still felt that initial pull toward adolescent medicine and was able to spend extra elective time with an OHSU adolescent medicine physician, Dr. Wayne Sells, who steered her to a number of influential rotations, including working in a clinic for homeless teenagers in Portland called Outside In. "I thought that was one of the coolest things ever," she said. While it was near the end of her third year of residency, and thus very late in the application process, Dr. Sells still encouraged her to apply for an adolescent medicine fellowship.

This was prior to the National Resident Matching Program (NRMP) system, so she called every board-certified fellowship program in the country (twelve at the time) to inquire about openings. The University of Rochester (UR) was one such program that was recruiting fellows. "I remember having a conversation with Dr. Rich Kreipe at the U of R who was extremely enthusiastic and passionate about adolescent health," she said. Dr. Kreipe, the fellowship program director at the time, invited her to interview and even used his frequent flyer points for her to do so, as traveling from the West Coast to the East Coast would have been financially prohibitive. She immediately fell in love with the program and the people and instantly knew this was where she wanted to spend the next three years.

As a fellow, Dr. Yussman was part of the Leadership Education in Adolescent Health (LEAH) program, which was extremely robust during the time of her fellowship, from 2000 to 2003. Even though she arrived in Rochester without knowing anyone, she says the LEAH program introduced her to a wonderful multidisciplinary group of people her age who had similar interests. "We created this really strong bond of young adults who really loved adolescent health," she said. She received fantastic training and had the added opportunity to pursue her Master of Public Health (MPH) degree, which she says gave her the background and confidence to have success with scholarly activity.

As the end of her fellowship neared, Dr. Yussman was disappointed that Rochester did not have any job opportunities available, but this gave her a wonderful networking experience of interviewing throughout the country. She was strongly leaning toward accepting a position at the University of Michigan in Ann Arbor when her boyfriend at the time, now husband, proposed to her. He was from Rochester and had just started his own local business, limiting his ability to leave the area. Dr. Yussman spoke with Drs. Elizabeth McAnarney and Kreipe, who were able to piece together a full-time job for her—fifty percent of her time at the University of Rochester in the Division of Adolescent Medicine, and fifty percent at an inner-city teen clinic, Threshold Center for Alternative Youth Services.

Serving as the medical director at Threshold remains one of Dr. Yussman's proudest roles. "We had a fabulous group of people who were working with some very under-resourced teenagers and young adults who were incredibly grateful for the care that we provided," she said. This ambulatory clinic served patients between the ages of twelve and twenty-five years and offered primary care services, as well as strong reproductive health care. Threshold was located directly on a bus line and was walkable for many adolescents and young adults. Parental consent for reproductive health care was not required, which made this care confidential, and the clinic offered evening and Saturday hours to help increase access. Unfortunately, after a series of ownership changes and eventual financial issues, Threshold's teen services were significantly decreased as it was finally subsumed under another agency. Over the years, Dr. Yussman has continued her work with community programs, including serving as the senior pediatrician for Hillside Family of Agencies, where she consults with the nurse practitioners providing direct medical care to teens in their residential programs. As fellowship program director, she encourages and enables her fellows to have community experiences through the wide-ranging, diverse rotations offered to them.

Dr. Yussman became the fellowship program director in 2010 and is proud of the program's growth. In the past twenty years, the community clinical elective offerings, many of which are unique to Rochester's program, have at least doubled. Oftentimes it is fellow interest that generates new electives, which Dr. Yussman and the program enthusiastically facilitate. "I think that helps fellows recognize all of the diverse options for positions they have after graduation; that is, they may or may not want to incorporate some similar programs into their future employment as faculty members," she said.

Dr. Yussman is also particularly proud of her community outreach work with the Rochester City School District (RCSD). She served as the collaborating physician and medical director for several RCSD schools, including East, Franklin, and Douglass High Schools, until the Nurse Practitioners Modernization Act for New York State ended the need for that role. However, the University of Rochester's School of Nursing oversees two of the city's school-based health centers (SBHC), and because of the strong collaboration Dr. Yussman built with the nursing staff at these schools, she was able to continue a relationship and expand the work they had started. In 2016, when East High School was at risk for closure due to poor school performance, the school opened a request for proposals for agency collaboration to help make improvements at the school and ultimately improve student outcomes. Dr. Yussman and the School of Nursing's Kim Urbach, PNP, who directs the

SBHCs, assembled a group of providers and community members, brainstormed services they could improve, and applied for and received six years of grant funding from the Greater Rochester Health Foundation (GRHF).

Dr. Yussman's and Ms. Urbach's team established three major initiatives: (1) initiating universal sexually transmitted infections (STIs) screening for any student who comes to the health center; (2) improving the school's free breakfast program, which was being underutilized; and (3) screening all middle school students for adverse childhood experiences (ACEs) and offering subsequent in-school group therapy for those who score the highest (the most adverse experience). They saw remarkable results. They were able to find and treat an overwhelmingly higher number of STIs, helping to decrease the burden of these diseases in the student population. Through changing bus schedules and allowing students to pick up a grab-and-go-style breakfast to eat in their first period classes, they saw the number of students choosing to have breakfast double. Both of these programs are self-sustaining and no longer dependent on grant funding.

In-school group therapy is an offering of which Dr. Yussman and the group are particularly proud. "The goal is to work on resilience and coping skills, with the thought that if we can improve students' resilience, then they can improve in many ways and have the best possible future and long-term outcomes," she said. "It has been incredible to see the kind of responses we have had, particularly from students, but also parents, teachers, and administrators." This program will also be self-sustaining after they transition its administration to the school social workers.

In 2017, another leadership opportunity came to Dr. Yussman when she was offered the position of interim division chief, followed by appointment to be division chief in 2019. "I feel that I'm a pretty humble person at baseline and while I wanted to do well and grow the field, I never thought 'I have to be fellowship director' or 'I have to be division chief,'" she said. "But as those opportunities arose, I was excited to be asked to do, or to be offered, those things." She laughs, recalling the time when she first graduated from fellowship and there was not a single job available to her in Rochester compared with where she now stands. "It's what I share with my fellows, too—you feel like you have these specific plans, but there are twists and turns that you don't expect, or opportunities that arise to which you're going to say yes or no. I'm so appreciative of the exciting opportunities that come my way," she said.

As division chief, she has participated in the growth of adolescent medicine in the region beyond eating disorders. While she says that the treatment of eating disorders remains important work, her team has also been able to expand their other clinical services, including that of gender health and reproductive health. In under ten years, the gender health program has expanded from a panel of single-digit patients to nearly 575, less than 100 patients fewer than the division's longstanding eating disorder program in the academic year ending in June 2021. "If you build it, they will come," she said. Above all, she is extremely proud of the team they have assembled, which she says is more like a family.

Reflecting on the history of the division and the leaders before her, she says, "I think of all of our mentors who helped start adolescent medicine, particularly Dr. McAnarney and her incredible mentorship and strong leadership within the Department of Pediatrics, which has really helped elevate the Division of Adolescent Medicine and bring it to the forefront." She notes the legacies of Dr. McAnarney's Rochester Adolescent Maternity Program (RAMP) and Dr. Kreipe's eating disorder and LEAH programs, and she remains impressed that Rochester had one of the first board-certified fellowship programs in adolescent medicine. She tries not to take for granted the international leaders that are right down the hallway and says, "It's really exciting to be able to get that historical perspective from them and also to use that knowledge to help move the field forward."

Dr. Yussman has witnessed many changes in the field during her time in practice, from the growth of services like gender health, to the Affordable Care Act that allowed adolescents to remain on their parents' insurance until age twenty-six, something that had a huge and positive influence on young adult access to health care. She knows challenges remain in the future, especially in light of the events that took place surrounding the COVID-19 pandemic, including mental health risks, racial disparities, unemployment, and substance abuse. "I think there are so many issues that are being magnified right now that our teenagers are going to need a lot more support at home, at school, and in clinical settings," she said. Another challenge she believes the field will continue to face is that of electronic medical records and ensuring confidentiality for teenagers, something that has become increasingly difficult and nuanced with the advancement of technology. However, she remains optimistic, as she says she has seen the field grow and improve over the years—from the improved focus on LGBTQ+ youth and diversity to continuous new research on adolescent neurodevelopment and an emphasis on interprofessional teams that include the patient at the forefront—"I definitely feel that adolescent health has improved," she said.

Dr. Yussman is a valued mentor, educator, advocate, and leader in the division and the Rochester community. She has developed the fellowship program further and the division's clinical services, continuing the strong legacy of adolescent medicine at the University of Rochester, the greater community, Western New York region, and beyond. With her remarkable leadership skills and her high intellectual, professional, and personal achievement, she leads through example. Her colleagues in the Division of Adolescent Medicine, the Department of Pediatrics, and the greater Rochester community look to Dr. Yussman to provide a guiding light for optimal care of adolescents and young adults, education of future health professionals, and creation of questions in adolescent medicine, all of which are critical to the current and future health of adolescents and young adults.

ABOUT THE AUTHORS

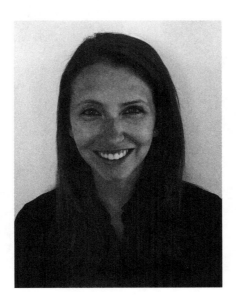

MEGHAN PLOG received her BA in English literature from DePauw University and her MS in Education from the University of Rochester's Warner School of Education. She feels fortunate to have worked with the remarkable Division of Adolescent Medicine at the University of Rochester during her time as an Administrator in the Department of Pediatrics, particularly serving as Program Coordinator for the Adolescent Medicine Fellowship program from 2015 to 2019. In 2019 she relocated to St. Louis, Missouri, where she began working in the Department of Pediatrics at Washington University School of Medicine.

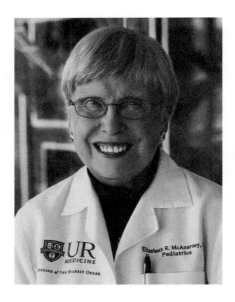

ELIZABETH R. MCANARNEY, MD, has been a member of the University of Rochester Medical Center for over fifty-five years. She is a Distinguished University Professor and Chair Emerita of the Department of Pediatrics. Her research in pediatrics is based in Adolescent Medicine.